RETHINKING CANCER

NON-TRADITIONAL APPROACHES to the THEORIES, TREATMENTS and PREVENTION of CANCER

RUTH SACKMAN

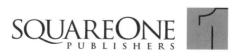

SQUAREONE
PUBLISHERS

The information and advice contained in this book are based upon the research and the personal and professional experiences of the author. They are not intended as a substitute for consulting with a health care professional. The publisher and author are not responsible for any adverse effects or consequences resulting from the use of any of the suggestions, preparations, or procedures discussed in this book. All matters pertaining to your physical health should be supervised by a health care professional. It is a sign of wisdom, not cowardice, to seek a second or third opinion.

COVER DESIGNER: Phaedra Mastrocola
IN-HOUSE EDITOR: Elaine Kennedy
TYPESETTER: Gary A. Rosenberg

Square One Publishers
115 Herricks Road
Garden City Park, NY 11040
(516) 535-2010 • (877) 900-BOOK
www.squareonepublishers.com

Library of Congress Cataloging-in-Publication Data

Sackman, Ruth.
   Rethinking cancer : non-traditional approaches to the theories, treatments, and prevention of cancer / Ruth Sackman.
      p. ; cm.
   Includes bibliographical references and index.
   ISBN 0-7570-0093-2 (pbk.)
1. Cancer–Alternative treatment.
   [DNLM: 1. Neoplasms—therapy. 2. Complementary Therapies.
3. Neoplasms—prevention & control. QZ 266 S121r 2003] I. Title.
RC271.A62 S335   2003
616.99'406—dc22

                                      2003016781

Printed in the United States of America

10   9   8   7   6   5   4

Contents

Dedicated to my husband Leon
and my daughter Arlene

Acknowledgments

I t is difficult for me to express in words how deeply I appreciate all the people who helped me on the long circuitous path that has led to this book. They gave generously and patiently of their time and expertise because they believed in the importance of communicating the information I have acquired during the course of my thirty plus years as president of FACT.

First let me thank Irving Wexler, Ph.D. in English Literature, author of several books of poetry and fiction, who was instrumental in helping me, especially in the initial stages of this work. He created an outline and worked with me through the basics of getting my thoughts on paper, as well as always being there for questions of clarity, continuity, syntax, proofreading, etc. and all with wonderful energy and enthusiasm. I am also so grateful to Consuelo Reyes, Trustee on the FACT Board of Directors, who spent countless hours transferring the manuscript to the computer, which infinitely simplified the tasks of editing, proofreading, etc. She also was a godsend coming to my rescue whenever my computer skills reached a dead end! Heartfelt thanks to Josephine Coppa, who was absolutely invaluable in reading the manuscript and making suggestions and finally getting the text into professional book form. I owe a profound debt of gratitude to Stephanie Tevonian, a professional book designer, who took time out of her extremely hectic schedule to design the pages of the book in the present very readable, attractive style. And finally, special thanks to all the FACT Board members—Martin Fall, Rhoda Koeppel, Nicholas Daflos, Corinne Loreto, Consuelo Reyes and my husband, Leon Sackman— for their loving, consistent encouragement and support because they believed so strongly in the importance of bringing this book to the public.

Finally, I feel these acknowledgements would not be complete if I did not express my gratitude to my teachers, the numerous highly qualified clinicians worldwide, the forefathers of today's health movement, who shared their invaluable insights and experience with me. I was fortunate that they passed on their experience so unselfishly because they understood the value of an organization like FACT. They were healers in the true sense and I was the beneficiary of their voluminous knowledge.

My first contact was with Dr. William Donald Kelley, a recovered cancer patient, who developed an individualized, metabolic system of host repair by investigating the field in his effort to treat himself. I met him at a convention in California and invited him to speak at a FACT meeting in New York. We had ample time to visit before and after the meeting to discuss his work in depth. Subsequently, we made many referrals to Dr. Kelley and had an unusual opportunity to work with him, his patients and their doctors. This is a way in which we collected in depth data about a doctor's work.

The next person to whom I am grateful for adding to my education was Ebba Waerland. We met when she was already retired, in her eighties, living in Switzerland and overcoming the damage from an automobile accident. She and her husband, Are, owned and directed a clinic in Sweden. The Waerland System, which was a method of prevention and restoration, was adopted by about forty clinics in Europe. Many Europeans used a stay at the clinics for a yearly restoration. I had a very productive association with this wonderful lady via mail and telephone. It was through her that I met Dr. Karl Aly.

Dr. Aly, now retired, was the director of the original Waerland Clinic which Ebba Waerland referred to as the "Mother Clinic." This is a 90 bed facility in Sunnansjo, Sweden which is still serving patients. Dr. Aly's knowledge about nutrition and physiology was incomparable and I, fortunately, was the avid recipient of this information which he so generously provided.

Dr. Bernard Jensen, an expert in iridology and nutrition based on clinic work, ran the Hidden Valley Health Ranch in Escondido, California. He and I enjoyed a long friendship, as was true with many of the people who were practicing biologically sound healing methods. I became the grateful trustee of Dr. Jensen's 60 years of knowledge. What an outstanding reward!

Dr. Max Warmbrand practiced Naturopathy for over 60 years in Norwalk, Connecticut. He introduced me to many of his recovered patients which provided me with a wonderful opportunity to learn about his work first hand. We also spent many productive hours of conversation over frequent dinners which we enjoyed at Farm Food, a vegetarian restaurant in

New York City. How many students of physiology and natural healing can have this personal relationship with their teachers?

Dr. Jesse Mercer Gehman, who was the head of an international health organization, spent many an evening with me on the telephone discussing natural healing. He had written frequently for a number of health publications and had an extensive file of articles. When our discussion related to something he had written, he would follow up by sending the printed item. It was a learning opportunity which is impossible to duplicate.

Dr. Leo Roy, a physician and surgeon, came to a FACT convention in New York City and introduced himself to me. Our relationship which lasted many years was most rewarding. Dr. Roy spent 6 months working with Dr. Max Gerson at his clinic in Nanuet, New York. (Dr. Gerson, although trained traditionally, was a pioneer in biologically sound healing.) Another aspect of Dr. Roy's expertise was his motivation to investigate every realistically sound health restoration idea wherever it existed. He traveled abroad and throughout the United States and Mexico to acquire the broad, in-depth knowledge he applied in serving his patients.

I feel I was favored by the gods to have had this fruitful association with these outstanding people whose clinic experience is unmatched today. Because I have had these experienced people as my teachers, I feel obliged to pass on their gift to me through this book.

Foreword

I t is an honor to introduce this book by my longtime friend Ruth Sackman. It is a distillation of the practical wisdom Ruth has acquired through her many years of counseling and guiding people with cancer. Although a layperson, Ruth's approach to cancer is scientific in the true sense of the word, based on a combination of keen observation and clear thinking, with no prejudices or agendas to muddy the waters.

These capacities for free and unbiased observation and thinking lie at the heart of science—how greatly they are needed today!

Ruth has been a forerunner of the current trend of renewed interest and participation in medicine and healing by consumers. Any intelligent, practical person motivated to serve one's fellow human being and willing to follow the discipline of clear thinking could draw much inspiration from Ruth's example.

Specialized knowledge is of great value, but healing is too important to be left to the experts alone. A healthy system has checks and balances. In medicine these can be provided by the participation and the unique perspective of the informed and concerned consumer.

But something else is needed to get our ailing medical system, and with it the health of our citizens, on the right track. What is needed is a remedy for the curious tunnel vision that afflicts most of us today, expert and consumer alike.

Ruth is remarkably free of this problem, making this book doubly valuable. This tunnel vision is what biologist Craig Holdrege calls "object-thinking."* This object-thinking seems to belong to our modern worldview.

In medicine, it is the tendency to view an illness as a sharply defined object, as an alien "other" with a life and agenda of its own that has seized

---

*Holdrege, C. 1996 *Genetics & the Manipulation of Life: The Forgotten Factor of Context.* pp. 51–52. Hudson, New York: Lindisfarne Press.

hold of us and with whom we are one. When we look at cancer through the lens of object-thinking, we see only the tumor, and not the process that created it. We see the tumor as a foreign object, a self-created thing, and we ignore the context out of which the tumor arose. We forget that we ourselves are the context. As Ruth makes clear in this book, a tumor doesn't appear in a vacuum, it is a product of the entire physiological and psychological history of its individual host resulting in a breakdown in body chemistry which allows the production and accumulation of malignant cells. Object-thinking focuses only on the malignant cell itself, and naturally seeks the cause of cancer within the cell. This is tunnel vision. Cells depend on the conditions of the body's inner biochemical environment just as plants depend on outer environmental conditions of soil, water and light. In both cases the context is all important.

This context is the patient and his or her own particular life journey, which has led to greater and greater physiological imbalance in the body until the breaking point is reached and the tumor appears. Ruth points to the long history of disturbed homeostasis preceding most diagnoses of cancer.

In what she calls the overriding theme of the book, Ruth emphasizes that no cancer can be properly treated merely by destroying the cancer cells. A successful long-term result will always depend on restoring homeostasis and on repairing the breakdown in body chemistry which produced the malignant cells in the first place and allowed them to gain a foothold in the body.

Just how this repair and restoration are achieved, and if they are achievable, will differ in each individual host. There are no magic bullets, no panaceas in cancer treatment. This book includes many helpful, practical guidelines and enlightening case histories, all the time emphasizing that success in preventing and treating cancer can never be reduced to a formula and needs the guidance of a health professional with practical experience.

Cancer is a life-threatening, life-changing crisis that demands the utmost of our capacities for courage, self-knowledge, growth and change.

Cancer can be a reminder of our life's meaning and purpose. It is a frightening adversary that, with the grace of God and a lot of hard work on our part, I believe can become a friend bestowing blessings.

Philip Incao, M.D.

Introduction

For a number of years many of my associates at the Foundation for Advancement in Cancer Therapy (FACT), doctors, friends, members and others in the health field, have urged me to write a book that would systematically document all the knowledge I had acquired about the biological approach to cancer, health and disease. It was their feeling that what I had learned through my extensive experience as president of FACT should be made readily available to the largest possible number of patients and practitioners. I was extremely reticent about introducing a revolutionary concept of cancer to a population accustomed to the present concept of cancer as an inviolate truth. Letting go of established ideas can be very difficult.

Even so, periodically, I had promised myself to take off the considerable time that would be necessary to think through and carry out such an ambitious undertaking. For, indeed, I had felt all along that there was a great and growing need to help a broader spectrum of people learn about biological approaches to cancer treatment and other degenerative ailments that have developed over many decades, than was possible through the often hectic daily operations of the foundation. More than that, I had been troubled not only by a lack of popular understanding of this important subject, but also by the enormous amount of misinformation that is now being disseminated under the banner of so-called "alternative therapies."

With these ends in mind, I spent a number of years compiling information. This book is based on my experiences, investigations, observations and conclusions gathered over the past 30 years on this subject. The outcome of this labor is this volume, *Rethinking Cancer: Non-Traditional Approaches to the Theories, Treatments and Prevention of Cancer.*

My colleagues and I at FACT firmly believe in the public's right to be fully informed about the biological approach to the restoration of health, non-toxic cancer therapies and alternatives to orthodox treatments for cancer. To help make this possible, I shall try to pass on to you, the reader, all of the considerable information about the biological concept of health care collected by FACT under unique conditions. I have acquired this knowledge through direct contact with many thousands of cancer patients, with many doctors (clinicians) who are practicing this therapeutic direction and my visits to the many clinics in Europe, Mexico and the United States. By bringing this in-depth material together in one place, I hope that it can be more effectively utilized by the practitioner, the patient and their family.

I cannot emphasize strongly enough that the purpose of this book is not to give advice or recommend specific procedures to anyone. My aim is, rather, to make available carefully scrutinized information based on my *years of experience.* Once he or she has acquired sufficient information, he or she should be in a position to make intelligent decisions as a medical consumer. Although I believe that the ultimate responsibility for getting well lies with the patient, I urge him or her to seek the help of a competent advisor.

It is not FACT's intent to discredit practitioners of standard medicine. Nor do we question the skill, sincerity or integrity of physicians. We have excellent relations and work cooperatively with qualified doctors in the United States, Canada, Europe and other areas of the world. Over the years FACT has given financial support to a number of biological investigations by men and women of science at established research institutions.

Actually, attitudes toward biological concepts on the part of many within the medical profession are much better today than they were even a short time ago. For example, we at FACT are beginning to find that information about cancer coming to us from conventional sources confirms what we have been saying to the cancer patient and the public-at-large for years. FACT has always considered a balanced metabolic program the backbone of biological therapy—*the nutrients in the food supply are the essential elements for building normal healthy cells.* More than a decade ago the National Cancer Institute established a department of diet and nutrition (now dissolved) and published a pamphlet with nutritional guidelines which is still available to the public, whereas, several decades ago conventional medicine negated any cancer/diet link. I am also pleased to note that the American Cancer Society, one of the major bastions of orthodox cancer therapies, held a seminar on the subject of nutrition and cancer. In these and many other ways, we think that the climate is moving—albeit far too slowly to be sure—toward acceptance of the biological repair system as a valid direction in cancer treatment.

The Concept of Biological Repair

How do FACT's views on cancer treatment differ from those held by traditional medicine? Briefly, the conventional approach believes that the tumor itself is, in effect, the disease and that cancer can be efficiently controlled by directing the therapy toward destroying the malignancy. The treatments most frequently used are radiation, chemotherapy, surgery and hormone inhibitors, or a combination of these procedures. Thus, the major focus of this traditional approach is *tumor destruction.*

We at FACT, on the other hand, support a concept of cancer as being a systemic malfunction which requires a biological repair. According to this concept, cancer cells are only a symptom of a dysfunction of the organism, resulting from a steady breakdown in the balance of body chemistry. Only by restoring the balance through safe and sound biological means can the disease be truly controlled. Conjointly, we believe that if given the proper support and a better lifestyle, the body's own inherent ability to repair itself could prevent cancer in the vast majority of cases. The major focus of the biological approach, therefore, is *host integrity.*

This is not a lay point of view, but an approach held by many practitioners over many decades who treated degenerative diseases by restoring the balance in body chemistry to its recovery potential through the use of biologically sound techniques—balanced nutrition and other forms of non-toxic, non-invasive therapies. After a thorough investigation of the writings of scientists and doctors, and close contact with many of them as well as with *recovered cancer patients,* I have concluded that these views offer the cancer patient an opportunity for a realistic, long-term recovery.

There exists a long list of highly competent practitioners—some going back to the latter part of the nineteenth century—who treated disease by optimizing the body's ability to repair itself. There was Max Gerson, M.D., a man who was lauded by Dr. Albert Schweitzer as "one of the most eminent geniuses in medical history." Other notable doctors include: John H. Tilden, M.D.; Benedict Lust, M.D.; I. Duncan Bulkley, M.D.; John Harvey Kellogg, M.D.; Are Waerland, Ph.D.; Norman W. Walker, D.Sci.; William

Howard Hay, M.D.; Henry Bieler, M.D.; Max Warmbrand, N.D.; Andrew Ivy, M.D.; William Frederick Koch, M.D.; Julian Baldor, M.D.; Sir William Arbuthnot Lane, M.D.; as well as many others.

Today immunotherapeutic techniques are recognized as a valid treatment in medical circles. Drs. Andrew Ivy and William Frederick Koch were supporters of immunotherapy early in the twentieth century. It is important to note that practitioners came to similar conclusions while working independently of one another—some in the United States, others in Europe and elsewhere. This phenomenon is evidence that helps to validate the biological repair approach to cancer treatment.

Hunger for Health

Today the public's hunger for health information is enormous. To a greater degree than ever before, people are deeply concerned about a wide range of factors that might affect their well-being: the air they breathe, the foods they eat, the water they drink, and the quality of medical care they receive. To answer this thirst for knowledge, a flood of material is now available on every conceivable health question—from environmental problems to dietary regimes, from cancer to high blood pressure, from meditation techniques to proper breathing, from spinal alignment to temporomandibular joint (TMJ) adjustment. A glance at the bookshelf in any health food or book store will confirm that publications relating to health are among the most saleable commodities.

What accounts for this tremendous surge of interest in matters dealing with health? In my opinion the reason for this interest is—to put it bluntly—the increasing sickness of our population. In alarming numbers people are not well—and I am referring not only to the virtual epidemic of cancer, but to every other form of degenerative illness as well. I came across a book written by a German scientist, Dr. Johannes Kuhl, which documents the total number of individuals who are being treated for all kinds of major degenerative diseases. Let me assure you that the statistics in this book make for pretty grim reading!

Too many people who depend on conventional doctoring are not getting good results. They are discovering that the medications and other treatments they have been receiving are not restoring their health. These medications temporarily alleviate symptoms without getting at the underlying causes of the illness. Unfortunately, many of the medicines have side effects, and therefore, should be used only when absolutely necessary, not just to avoid minor discomfort.

Today there are simply too many sick people. Nature didn't create a situation where so many human beings are doomed to suffer from all kinds of major ailments such as cancer, and to die in a slowly deteriorating, often agonizingly painful process, or linger on for years before death often thankfully comes. This condition was created by man.

We are no longer living in biblical times, when the lifespan allotted to humankind was threescore and ten. In our modern advanced technological age we ought to be able to live out a far longer and *healthier* lifespan. As a matter of fact I recently read a statement by a doctor in which he estimated that the average human being should live to be over a hundred years of age. Yet, only a small handful of people achieve that milestone. As far as the majority of the population is concerned, life expectancy is a little over seventy. Despite the vast amounts of money that we here in the United States spend on health, and all of the so-called medical miracles, our nation ranges about *twenty-fourth* in the world in the life expectancy rate.

When we look at the cancer statistics, then, of course, the picture is truly disquieting. Today the cancer incidence, according to the American Cancer Society, has risen to an estimated 1,334,100 new cases in 2003. In 1975 the insurance industry issued a statement to the effect that the cancer rate had risen by 5.2%. For a number of years previous to that, the rise in the rate had run somewhere around 1.3%. Instead of being alarmed by that tremendous increase, the U.S. Bureau of Statistics placed the figure at 3.2% by officially attributing the higher death rate to the flu epidemic of 1975. But the fact remains that those were *cancer patients* who died from the flu; they did so because of the extreme weakness brought about by the cancer condition. Too often death certificates read heart failure, renal failure, respiratory failure or malnutrition. No juggling of statistics, however, can alter the fact that cancer is at epidemic levels. The present research, in spite of the glowing media reports, is really no closer to a cure than it was 100 years ago. *The solution is probably too simple for scientific minds to conceive that this treacherous disease, cancer, needs to focus on cell production rather than cell destruction.* It's a simple concept but it is difficult for people to shift their focus from killing what they have believed to be deadly cancer cells.

But these cancer statistics are not the only evidence of the abysmal state of health in our nation. All one has to do is look at the number of hospitals, the crowded hospital beds, their huge staff of doctors, the incredible sums of money spent on medical care, and especially the amount of drugs distributed by the pharmaceutical companies.

Is it not surprising that people are more health conscious than ever before, that they are searching for better answers to their health problems, and turning in other directions for health care? Those of us who are associated with FACT are in a particularly good position to observe the steadily rising number of individuals who are choosing biological repair systems, not only to deal with cancer and other degenerative diseases, but as a way of life to maintain their well-being.

The Dangers of Misinformation

Though the rise in the level of health consciousness among so many Americans is heartening, it has its built-in problems too. In their eagerness for more information and for biologically sound alternative therapies, many people turn to what are misnamed "natural" or "holistic" cures— many of which have not undergone the long-term clinical experience which is essential in establishing validity. Unfortunately, there are far too many people seeking biological therapies and not enough competent practitioners. Because of this, a number of individuals on the periphery of the health movement, who have little more knowledge than the average person, presume to give others advice or even set themselves up in practice. Hopefully, this book may be of some service in discouraging such people from misguiding others. Restoring health is a complex process requiring the guidance of competent people.

Since many people find it lucrative to deal with those who are desperate for help, it is important for the health-seeker to be very discriminating. Even with the best of intentions, overzealous persons may offer recommendations based on their own personal, though limited, experience. The therapeutic approach that may have worked well for them may be entirely wrong for another individual. I cannot begin to emphasize enough the serious consequences that can result from incompetent information involving biological therapies. In the case of a cancer patient, incompetent information can be particularly hazardous.

Let me further illustrate why and how erroneous information can be harmful to one's health. Because of the limited number of resources supplying biologically sound service, too many people with a great deal of heart, but with too little skill and knowledge, are trying to help others correct their health problems. Invariably, they do not have the experience acquired from serving a wide variety of patients; nor do they have the opportunity for consistent feedback to provide effective service. They may, for example, advise people to make major nutritional changes. As we will see later on in this book, food is a *potent* healer. Changes in dietary regimes can provoke profound adjustments in body chemistry that can be quite disturbing—and dangerous—to the uninformed cancer patient. Under no circumstances, therefore, should an individual begin a new nutritional regime without first consulting an experienced practitioner or an organization such as FACT which can provide guidance or recommend a resource best suited to a person's needs.

Too often the assumption is made that because a doctor is sympathetic to the biological approach, he or she, therefore, has acquired adequate knowledge and clinical experience to guide a patient through the different therapies. Let me state here, unequivocally, that there is no way to validate the success or failure of a therapy without including the time factor. For some types of cancer this time factor may be as long as 6 to 10 years. A practitioner, for instance, can initiate a metabolic regime with excellent results for months or even a few years. The patient may feel better and continue to make good progress during that time. On this basis, the practitioner and patient assume that he or she has the universal answer to the cancer problem and very soon the patient begins to promote a prematurely evaluated therapy as a success story. However, a few years later there may be a complete breakdown—because it was actually a deficient or unsound system at the start. The time element is a crucial factor in evaluating the success of a biological therapy.

Sometimes well-meaning individuals recommend institutions to cancer patients without in-depth knowledge of the facility or how successful they are in treating cancer or if it is the correct choice for a particular patient's condition. As we have seen at FACT, this type of advice could lead patients to inappropriate therapies that seriously jeopardize their health.

There are also individuals writing "one size fits all" books. They may be writing purely on the basis of theory, interviews, or from a background of nothing but laboratory work with mice or other experimental animals. Since the work has not been tested on human beings, there is no way of assessing whether it is sound or unsound. Let us say, for example, that the book is about vitamins or other forms of supplementation. In setting forth a specific program of food supplements the author cannot possibly take into account the state of health or the particular needs of each individual reader. One person may need one kind of supplement and not another. If someone advises him to take supplementation that his body doesn't require, it may ultimately unbalance the system on the side of excess.

How, then, does one differentiate between accurate and misleading information? In large measure this is the purpose of this book: to provide you with carefully collected time-proven information from FACT.

About FACT

At this point I think it appropriate to discuss the organization which, for three decades, has been a rich repository for the information presented in this book. FACT, an international organization, has executive headquarters in New York City. The Foundation for Advancement in Cancer Therapy is a federally approved, tax-exempt, nonprofit organization which distributes information about cancer prevention and non-toxic cancer therapies. Our main goal is to change the direction of cancer treatment. In addition, FACT supports and funds biological and scientific nutritional investigations and works to eliminate carcinogenic substances from the environment. FACT was established specifically as a *lay* organization in order to insure freedom of expression without jeopardizing any individual's medical license.

Among its many activities, FACT publishes the journal, *Cancer Forum*, and offers a carefully selected and frequently updated list of books, articles and tape recordings. Some of this material is specifically for doctors and other health professionals. We have sponsored Cancer/Nutrition Conventions, bringing together experts in the health field. And, periodically, I have presented information on television and have conducted a cancer/nutrition series on radio.

Whenever possible we refer patients to practitioners whose services have consistently produced good results over a considerable period of time. Many of the patients maintain close contact with FACT for years, sometimes on a daily basis if they are going through troublesome periods. In our years of existence, we have served literally thousands of patients and their families. The feedback we get from them is an invaluable yardstick in helping us to determine the effectiveness of the therapies, as well as to evaluate the professionals who are producing the best work in the field of biological repair. When we refer patients to a doctor, we choose professionals with sound and broad clinical experience—someone who can follow the patient's progress carefully and make adjustments as needed. Someone, most importantly, who has treated patients with good results.

FACT is funded entirely by tax-deductible contributions. We maintain a standard: no one serving in the organization may have a vested interest in cancer; although members of the Board of Trustees are indeed well qualified to be health practitioners.

One of FACT's trustees, a woman with many years of experience in the health field, has studied iris analysis—a non-invasive form of diagnosis—at her own expense with Dr. Bernard Jensen, a master in this technique. The time and effort she put into this important training could have qualified her as a practitioner. She is a most competent individual who has helped people in whatever way she could, with no compensation whatsoever beyond the knowledge that she was serving cancer patients. This is typical of all of the trustees of FACT. Their dedication to our goals gave me the energy and inspiration to write this book.

A Personal Experience with Cancer

I have often been asked how I became involved, heart and soul, in an organization that has absorbed 5 to 6 days a week of my life, virtually twelve months a year for over 30 years. As the result of the agonizing experience of caring for a cancer victim in my own family, I came to FACT as did so many of my associates. Some time in early 1970 my daughter, Arlene, was diagnosed as having acute leukemia. As is true for so many people who seek help with cancer, my husband and I naively believed what we were told—that there was an 85% success rate using chemotherapy for leukemia—certainly a high percentage. At that time we felt pretty certain, actually, that this young woman of twenty-nine was not that ill and should be one of the 85% who were supposed to recover. We discovered the hard way that the image we had of the success of this traditional cancer therapy was simply not what people have been led to believe. In time, one finds that the 85% recovery rate is temporary—sometimes it is only a brief remission. One learns, too, what the term remission means: it is only a respite for the patient which can be as short as a day or two or as long as a few years. Ultimately, as we discovered, the acute leukemia patient dies, as did my daughter.

Later we came to understand that remission means one thing to conventional medicine and another thing to lay people—even to highly knowledgeable people like us. For most doctors, success is measured in survival time—even adding a few months to the average survival time for a particular form of cancer is hailed as an accomplishment. Statistically, the concept of a "cure" refers only to a five-year survival period. This means that some forms of cancer, notably Wilms tumor, skin cancer and Hodgkin's can be managed for at least five years. More recently breast cancer has been added to the list, but only because improved diagnostic techniques make earlier detection possible. This merely starts the clock earlier. The five-year survival period is rare in acute leukemia, and for some other types of cancer, there is minimal or short-term survival. So you can see, the overall cancer situation is really very bleak.

When my daughter, Arlene, was released from the hospital, she was sicker than when we first brought her in. All of the hopeful words she had heard that had made her feel comfortable about submitting to chemotherapy suddenly had no value. In desperation, when we saw that Arlene was not responding to the therapy, we began to probe in every possible direction. First, we devoured all kinds of written material that was related to cancer—from the medical libraries, *Reader's Digest*, *Life Magazine*, the newspapers, everywhere. And now that we were asking the doctor harder questions about Arlene's condition, he became evasive. Actually, he avoided us because he didn't have an answer to our queries.

At this point I called a friend who had taken an entirely different path to cure an ovarian tumor that had dropped her hemoglobin to the low level of 4.5 because of constant bleeding. Because of some traumatic experience in her life, she was terrified of surgery. Due to this intense phobia, she found a practitioner who placed her, instead, on a nutritional regime which stopped the bleeding in about three weeks. Her blood count, which had been dangerously low, began to return to normal.

Fortunately for us, her doctor was still practicing and, when we brought Arlene to see him, he was able to make a tremendous improvement in her situation by using a balanced nutritional program. Unfortunately, however, we were all working under severe handicaps. We were unfamiliar with the doctor's health program and he was unable to be frank with us without jeopardizing his license, or to utilize hospital facilities to carry out his therapeutic system properly. After about ten months, Arlene's condition became complicated—not due to the form of therapy he was using—but as a result of the disastrous effects of the chemotherapy administered earlier.

Given this situation, we panicked, Arlene panicked, and the doctor felt that he did not have the right to tell us to continue on the therapeutic regime. Because of the political climate in medicine, the responsibility for staying on the biological program had to be the patient's. Had we known then what we know now, we would have realized that we should, indeed, have stayed with this biological therapy and taken our chances. The system had proven that it could work. Perhaps it should have been given more of a chance to overcome the toxicity of chemotherapy. And if it had failed, at least it would have failed using a path that *could* have saved Arlene's life. Death certainly would have occurred with the conventional system, as indeed it did.

Instead, we submitted to our panic and Arlene went back to the hospital. There, without my knowledge or consent since she was not a minor (although the law might consider her legally incompetent because she was desperate), the oncologist started her again on chemotherapy. From then on it was all downhill. Like so many others in the same circumstances, we still clung to the hope that Arlene would be one of the 85% who recovered.

After Arlene passed away and we had somewhat recovered from the period of unbelievable agony and shock, we began to assess what had really happened. Since we had experienced some success with the biological approach in repairing her body chemistry—despite the damage done by the chemotherapy—we knew that a biologically sound system induced a potent response. We then found that there was an organization of people who were already discussing and using other concepts of cancer therapy. Ultimately, we discovered that there was a whole range of non-toxic therapies (to be discussed in a later chapter) that were on a separate track from conventional procedures.

We began to investigate the long history of doctors and scientists who had developed a body of theory and practice around the concepts of biological repair—the idea that the human system has great capacity to heal itself if there is cooperation, rather than interference, with its natural processes. Because this approach ran counter to the established view of cancer therapy, it had not been given the fair-minded investigation it deserved, even though there was good clinical history on record—case records of patients who had successfully navigated the process of biological repair and were alive and well many years after the original diagnosis. Unfortunately, neither the government nor the medical establishment has up to this time carried on a dialogue with those who have *long clinical* experience with this biological approach.

Some time later my husband and I opened up discussions with a group of individuals who believed, as we did, that the non-toxic way of handling health problems did warrant further investigation. Among this group were those who had lost a loved one to cancer and somehow been exposed to biologically sound ideas, as well as two cancer patients who chose a biological direction instead of conventional therapy. Instead of letting our tragic experience rest where it was, we decided to turn it into something that would help cancer patients who wished to use non-toxic therapies and sought the right to make their own choices. Out of this pioneer group was born the organization now called FACT.

Looking back now, I can see that it was stubbornness in my psychological make-up that motivated my decision to become an integral part of FACT. There was something about the whole process of Arlene's illness that was unreal. "This can't be. This is not supposed to happen. We can't allow our daughter's life to slip away without a fight. There must be a better way." These are the thoughts that go through stricken parents' minds when their child is dying of cancer. It is as though we said: "This tragic situation has got to stop—not only for our own, but for all children." We just knew then that we had the responsibility to pursue every direction that could offer a cancer patient hope. If the things we had learned from our bitter experience turned out to be invalid, well, at least these biological concepts had been given a chance to be proven right or wrong. But to negate this opportunity was—in our opinion—unconscionable.

I don't often use strong language, but I sincerely believe that to ignore one's obligation under these circumstances—with cancer at epidemic proportions and in view of the lack of success of conventional treatments—is really obscene, a violation of the human spirit. As I have already pointed out, over the years, the attitude of conventional practitioners has changed for the better, but at one time, not too far back, hostility to natural healing concepts was fierce. Despite the fact that they had helped many patients correct long-standing health problems, one doctor had to spend more than a million dollars in a court action defending his therapeutic approach and others spent time in jail because of their unorthodox ideas and practices.

Even today the cancer patient who wants to use a non-toxic treatment for his or her illness often has to travel far from home at considerable expense. This burden needs to be alleviated. The patient should have access to a doctor in his or her community, near to family, and with the cost borne by whatever health insurance he or she carries. Anything less is a violation of human rights.

There is beginning to be a meeting of minds with some doctors and scientists. With a sincere dialogue and proper research, the biological approach to cancer can prove its ability to achieve excellent results. I think the time is now to give the biological concept of curing cancer serious consideration.

Hopefully, this will happen rapidly. Until that time, however, organizations like FACT will still be needed to provide support for cancer victims, and a book like this will have to provide well-researched information which is still so difficult to find elsewhere.

1. Toward an Understanding of Health and Disease

When one tugs at a single thing in nature,
he finds it attached to the rest of the world.
—JOHN MUIR, NATURALIST

Quoting the bleak cancer statistics in this opening chapter is not meant to frighten people; its purpose is to show why this book is needed and hopefully be helpful in making a decision if there is a cancer diagnosis. This book offers what I feel is a long overdue and very different concept of cancer and cancer treatment.

"Cancer is one of the most frightening words in our language." So begins an important book on this subject written by a group of distinguished scientists and physicians under the auspices of the New York Academy of Sciences.

As the above publication, *Cancer and the Worker*, so graphically notes, there is good reason for the dread which the mere mention of this disease strikes in the hearts of so many. "At the present rate, three out of every ten Americans now living," the book continues, "will eventually have cancer. It can be expected to strike in two of every three families." Since the book was published, the statistics have changed dramatically and not for the better.

According to the authors, 351,000 Americans died of cancer in 1973. In 1974 deaths had climbed to 357,000; in 1975 to 364,000 (1000 per day). In 1977, the year the book appeared, the incidence of cancer deaths had reached 370,000—*one every two and a half minutes.*

Over 30 years later, despite media reports of progress, the situation is worse. In 2003, according to the American Cancer Society, 1 of 3 women received a cancer diagnosis; the figure for men was 1 of 2. Do we wait until it's 1 out of 1 before we change direction?

Usually, 50% of cancer patients do not survive for five years. One must also consider that these staggering figures do not include the additional number of persons who died of cancer but whose deaths were officially attributed to other causes such as malnutrition, heart failure or flu.

We are told "the cancer rate continues to go up steadily" despite the hundreds of millions of dollars that the government spends annually on its so-called "war on cancer." We need only look at the number of Americans in 2000—over 1,000,000 who found out they had cancer—to see that the warning sounded in this book continues to be tragically confirmed.

In one sense it is very valuable to be reminded by an influential group in the scientific and medical community that traditional forms of therapy have failed dismally to stem the tide of cancer. In another sense, however, the continued recital of bleak statistics—without providing a hopeful alternative—can only further contribute to the feeling of despair which permeates most people's attitudes toward this disease.

I have a great deal of respect for the skill and compassion of the medical profession as a whole and the highly qualified research and theoretical advances which have produced present-day cancer treatment. But it must be admitted that traditional treatments have failed to halt this scourge, and no solution to the cancer problem appears to be on the horizon in orthodox circles. If we at FACT thought that current therapies were effective, there would be no point to our existence, nor would research have to be supported by such massive assistance from government and private agencies. Based on positive experiences over the last 30 years, I believe that the concept of host repair using biologically-sound systems, which is the focus of this book, should be regarded as a significant and valid approach to the prevention, control and cure of cancer. It seems to me, therefore, that what is needed is a greater understanding of the basic principles underlying this biological approach to health and disease. Such a clarification will be helpful, not only to the practitioner and cancer patients who are already using biological therapies, but to anyone who is seeking a different pathway toward maintaining health, preventing cancer and prolonging life.

WHAT DOES HEALTH MEAN?

To begin with, we at FACT define health from the "total person" perspective. That is to say, the human body was designed by Nature as a unified whole in which all parts work together to achieve a balanced, fully coordinated functioning organism. Are Waerland, Ph.D., the originator of a system of health restoration which was the basis for establishing many health clinics in Europe, has described this interrelation of the human body as follows: "By means of the blood and nervous system, all the different organs and minutest parts of the body are bound together in an exquisitely adjusted homogeneous cell community, in which, normally, everything functions in normal harmony. A disturbance in any one part affects the whole."

From this whole person viewpoint, good health, under ideal circumstances, is a condition in which the individual is sound in every aspect of his or her being—psychologically as well as physiologically. And this harmonious state of being can come about when we conduct our lives in accord with the biological rhythms of Nature. It requires, as we shall see, a life-style which includes:

- a biologically-sound nutritional regimen

- efficient elimination of body wastes

- sufficient exercise

- adequate sleep

- stress control

- proper body alignment

- normal breathing

- healthy glandular, digestive, enzymatic and circulatory function, etc.

A large order, but certainly achievable. The body appreciates good treatment and responds in kind.

Since the mind is as important as the body in maintaining health, the healthy individual strives to maintain, as much as possible, a positive emotional attitude and spiritual values which can give direction, fulfillment and meaning to life.

Admittedly, this state of well-being may not be easily attainable in our disease-ridden society where stress and anxiety are the rule rather than the exception, much of our food is chemically polluted and treated, and the environment in which we live is constantly bombarded with dangerous contaminants. In spite of these negative factors, many people manage to live long, disease-free lives and others recover from disease. Moreover, it is possible for many others, who are afflicted with major diseases like cancer, to look forward to healthy and productive lives.

I say this with a full awareness that controlling cancer is not easy but is unquestionably possible. It requires effort on the part of the patient in terms of time, knowledge and determination—as well as a therapeutic program that includes all the resources needed in order to effect a recovery.

Fortunately, humans have been endowed by Nature with a *remarkable self-healing* capacity which I like to refer to as our "bio-repair system." When this inherent repair ability is left intact (or when it is not interfered with) it can help prevent disease and restore the body's biological integrity when cancer or other degenerative diseases occur. The longer I am involved with cancer patients, the more amazed I am to see what marvelous instruments our bodies are and the tenacity of the body's drive to fight for survival even under the most difficult circumstances. I am convinced that if only we do not obstruct the body's healing effort, if only we do not abuse our bodies with destructive habits, we can go a long way toward preventing and conquering the whole range of degenerative diseases—cancer among them—which still afflict a large part of the human race.

At one of FACT's Annual Conventions, Leo Roy, M.D. expressed this idea so beautifully that I think it is worth quoting: "Nature has given us as a birthright a reservoir of vital, self-healing forces which are the source of our enormous recuperative powers. Anything that diminishes this life force—whether it be exhaustion, dead foods, fear, anger, tension—thereby diminishes the body's defenses against disease. Anything that enhances this life force—whether it be sun, rest, good food, positive thinking and feeling the joy of life—thereby renews the body's ability to repair itself."

If you are ill, you may discover for yourself that one of the most important aspects of your recovery is being able to listen to and heed the signals of your body. When it tells you that it is tired, rest or sleep. When you are tense or under severe stress, seek ways to relax. Eat only when you are hungry and relaxed. Watch for telltale signs that your wastes need to be eliminated. Listen well. It is the best way to help the human organism maintain good health and repair the biological breakdown which has brought about the disease in the first place.

WHAT DOES DISEASE MEAN?

Turning from health to disease, we know, of course, that conventional medicine deals with illness largely in terms of symptoms—tumor in the case of cancer, the aches and pains of arthritis, palpitations of high-blood pressure, gnawing pain of ulcers, etc. Rarely is much emphasis placed on causes such as the individual's destructive life patterns, poor food, lack of sleep and exercise, constitutional weaknesses or the damaging effects of the pollutants in our environment—all of which play a vital role in producing illness. For the most part "curing" disease allopathically consists of attempts to alleviate symptoms, generally by means of a vast variety of drugs, or when deemed necessary, by surgical intervention or other biologically unsound means. Should any of these treatments result in the disappearance of symptoms even for a short period of time—the disease is deemed to have been "cured," even though the causative factors behind the symptoms have not been dealt with at all.

Most of the time when people experience distress, such as a headache, they take an aspirin or other painkiller. When they can't fall asleep, they take a sedative. And when they visit a doctor for a more serious problem— like high blood pressure—the doctor often prescribes an even more potent drug to relieve the symptom. Unfortunately, drugs do not correct causes, so the real problem is buried. This is the kind of abuse that gets heaped upon the body over the years. Eventually the cumulative effect contributes to a serious disturbance or breakdown of the biological processes.

Disease is seen as an outward manifestation of a long-term process (often decades in the making) that involves a biological breakdown in the capability of the body as a whole to carry on its life functions normally. Often a degenerative disease, such as cancer, originates in more than one cause, instead of being the result of one contributing factor. When disease does strike, it can be overcome or controlled only by normalizing the causes—whether they be nutritional, emotional, environmental, structural, or a combination of causes. It isn't that the distressing symptoms are ignored. As a matter of fact, a sound system of biological repair often relieves aches, pains, exhaustion, constipation, gas, and other symptoms as the dysfunction causing them is restored to normal.

When the body repairs with the help of a sound biological regimen and once again functions harmoniously, disease and its symptoms can be expected to be eliminated, up to the optimum level possible for each individual.

WHAT IS A BIOLOGICAL BREAKDOWN?

At this point you may wonder what I mean by the term "biological breakdown" which is used often in this book and is central to an understanding of nontoxic biologically sound therapies. To clarify, I will touch on some of the specific areas that can contribute to this process and provide more in-depth information in ensuing chapters.

The human organism has many systems with distinct functions. Any one of them can manifest a malfunction for a variety of reasons—accidents, chemicals, stress, structural imbalances, nutritional deficiencies, drugs, serious illnesses, x-rays, lack of sleep, and any violation of Nature's indispensable requirements. Constant offenses and interferences which compromise normal body function can result in troublesome symptoms. Chronic disturbances, seemingly minor, repeatedly offending the natural process, can play havoc with the physiological function of the body causing a breakdown in body chemistry. Organs need to function at an adequate level in order to sustain an individual's well-being.

Max Gerson, M.D., author of *A Cancer Therapy: Results of Fifty Cases*, and director of a clinic in Nanuet, New York, claimed that cancer resulted from a breakdown in liver function. Dr. William D. Kelley, author of the book *One Answer to Cancer*, claimed that cancer resulted from a breakdown in pancreatic function. I can agree with both of them. Cancer can be caused by a chronic dysfunction of any organs or bodily systems. An impairment can occur in the digestive, nervous, glandular, circulatory, elimination, immune, enzymatic, endocrine or any other system.

Structural imbalance can also impact on the normal function of the body. The nerve ends that relay instructions to our organs are located between the vertebrae of the spine. If these are blocked, the organs receive limited or unclear instructions.

THE WHOLE BODY CONCEPT

This complete interdependency of the human organs and their functions is at the heart of my discussion of biological breakdown. I want, therefore, to comment here on the role that conventional medicine has played in emphasizing the treatment of symptoms. It has been standard medical procedure to fragment the body into isolated parts and to treat those parts as though they were independent entities with no connection to the whole organism. Thus, if the kidney is damaged, the kidney specialist tends to treat that organ alone, without taking into consideration other biological factors. Since the body is an interrelated organism—one common bloodstream, endocrine system, nerve network, lymphatic system, waste elimination system and immune system—a breakdown in areas seemingly unrelated to the kidneys may be responsible for a kidney malfunction. The kidney functions within those interrelated systems as do all the organs.

In some cases health problems emanate from more than one direction, and have to be seen in a multi-causal light if the proper therapy is to be chosen. The workings of the body are subtle and complex. The following example might help us understand.

Dr. Lothar Wendt and several colleagues have done extensive research—primarily published in German—on the effects of the overuse of proteins. Protein metabolism is incomplete when the pancreas cannot supply sufficient proteolytic enzymes needed to metabolize the excess ingestion of meat. Excess protein, they found, is stored around the periphery of the cells. Normally there would be a density of no more than 300 angstrom units (a minute unit of length equal to one ten-thousandth of a micron or one hundred-millionth of a centimeter, used in expressing the length of light waves), but excess protein can build up to a density of thousands of angstrom units. Because of this thick coating on the cells, absorption of an adequate supply of nutrients and oxygen is diminished. We know that if cells do not get sufficient nourishment and oxygen, homeostasis is compromised.

Many competent practitioners who use biological therapies advise pancreatic enzyme supplements as a means of breaking down excess protein. This again is an example of how one poorly functioning or overloaded organ—in this case, the pancreas—can have a damaging effect on the cellular level.

Another example of a cause of a biological breakdown is when breast cancer metastasizes to the bone. I have had some experience with a number of patients whose breast cancers had metastasized where it was finally determined by the practitioners that poor thyroid function was interfering with the utilization of calcium. I can theorize that, under these circumstances, the body was draining calcium from the bones in its effort to supply the blood with this much-needed element. The cause of thyroid malfunctioning could be due to a hormonal imbalance. A book, *Natural Progesterone*, by John Lee, M.D., has documented how hormonal imbalance affects thyroid function. A thyroid dysfunction in turn affects calcium metabolism. The effect, no doubt, is analogous to menopause which usually results in osteoporosis, a condition related to bone loss. It is possible that breast cancer patients suffer from inadequate calcium metabolism. That could be the reason Dr. Max Gerson usually included thyroid supplementation in his cancer therapy.

In any discussion of a biological breakdown, we cannot omit the important role of the body's natural defense system (immune system) against disease. There is no one organ that functions as a center of immunity. The system is actually made up of a combination of many organs working together. As long as this unified defense system is active, it will make every effort to protect the body against the retention of any foreign material—and cancer cells are treated by the immune system as *foreign.*

We cannot ignore specialized cells such as the T-cells which are manufactured by the thymus gland to engulf foreign substances. But this is only one part of the complex system which makes resistance to disease possible. No one knows the intricacies of these processes yet, but enough is known to understand its impressive capability.

The immune system is not something that develops after a childhood disease and then protects against that disease only. This is a very narrow concept of immunity. A number of different organs and glands make up this system, including the thymus gland. But even the colon, liver, lymphatic system, lungs, skin and kidneys are integral to the immune process, since they help to eliminate toxic bioaccumulation (foreign waste products). And these waste products—if they are retained too long in the body, build up to a stressful level that creates a biochemical imbalance.

In the event that the organs of elimination are forced to overwork due to poor nutrition, smoking, chemical contaminants in the food and atmosphere, or stress, eventually they may become weakened to the point where they do not function well enough to maintain homeostasis. As a result of this breakdown, the immune system may no longer sufficiently clear the accumulated toxins from the cells, glands and bloodstream, thus depleting the immunological ability of the body to maintain a cancer-free environment.

The strength of any individual's immune defenses depends on many factors, including a predisposition. An interesting experiment done a number of years ago provides some evidence that a person's constitution determines to a large degree the effectiveness of his or her defense system. In this particular study, conducted by a group of Sloan-Kettering scientists, cancerous tissue from a human being was grafted onto the bodies of a number of volunteer prisoners. Some of the prisoners' bodies accepted the grafts; others rejected them.

The reason why some people accept foreign materials and others do not is very complex and revealing. What is relevant here, however, is that some of the subjects were able to reject the graft. Undoubtedly, it has to do with the fact that their immune systems were healthy at the time of the experiment, thus their immune responses were stronger than those of the others—clear evidence of the need to achieve and maintain competent host resistance. (I do not believe that the experiment created cancer in the individuals where the graft was accepted and produced a lump. The terrain was already vulnerable so the prisoners probably would have manifested symptoms eventually.)

I wouldn't want anyone to harbor the notion that all they have to do to remain healthy and cancer-free is to get an injection of an immunological substance. Alas, there is no magic immune bullet; first we have to improve the factors that contributed to the breakdown of the body's immune system.

WHY SOME SURVIVE—AND OTHERS DON'T

Considering the many abuses to which the average body is subjected over a lifetime and the various ways in which our systems can break down, the wonder is that so many of us maintain a state of reasonably good health. The only explanation for this lies in the extraordinary resilience and capacity for self-repair which Nature has bestowed upon us. We all know people who don't eat properly, smoke or drink, don't rest enough and otherwise pay scant attention to their health. In spite of that, they can have long, comfortable and disease-free lives. Without the abuses, it is possible they would live even longer.

The story that Norman Cousins tells in his bestselling book, *Anatomy of an Illness*, is a wonderful example of healing. The fact that he was able, in the course of a serious illness, to achieve a state of positive thinking and relaxation, is most likely the main factor in his recovery along with a strong constitution. There are people like him everywhere, whose sense of humor, optimism and sanity acts as a counterweight to the many destructive influences in our environment and to ourselves. When personal problems or serious emergencies arise, they can take them in stride and cope as best they can. In the same way, they treat world affairs lightly, confident that life will prevail come what may. It isn't that they are not concerned with serious problems such as environmental pollution, the possibility of war, the threat of dying or loss of employment; it is simply that they will not allow these problems—which have been with us for a long time—to stress them to the point where they get ill.

Very often we will find that this kind of individual enjoys life and is easily gratified by small pleasures. To a larger degree than you might think possible, a positive attitude is able to offset the harm of ingesting dreadful foods or breathing the polluted air and drinking the chemicalized water— problems that are by now almost universal. A relaxed attitude won't allow abnormal stress or emotional strains to interfere with the body's metabolism of food or elimination of waste. A healthy mind-set enables the body to derive maximum benefit from its innate healing capability.

Something that most people don't realize is that the human organism does not—believe it or not—need a great deal of food to provide the body with the essential nutrients to maintain health. It will extract the nourishment it needs and efficiently rid itself of whatever foreign substances need elimination provided that the body's systems have not broken down biologically beyond repair. For the most part, however, people with a reasonably sound constitution and a healthy lifestyle can continue in good health for many years, whereas, people with weak constitutions and the same lifestyle can succumb more readily to ill health.

As I write this I recall a question which a man asked me at a FACT Cancer/Nutrition convention: "How do you account for a two-year old child nurtured on the most perfect food there is, supposedly—breast milk—getting cancer as opposed to a sixty-year-old Bowery 'bum' who is drinking alcohol and picking cigarettes off the street, and still manages to survive and live without cancer?"

"There's something about that Bowery bum's constitution," I answered, "that is inherently strong and disease-resistant. The two-year-old can start at birth with a vulnerability to disease which has been acquired from its parents. That vulnerability is what leaves the child with a faulty defense system, so that even though the parents have provided the best of care, it couldn't prevent him or her from getting cancer." Therefore, some people have the good fortune to be blessed from birth with a sound constitution—while others do not. In order for the questioner not to feel responsible for his child's illness, I told him of my daughter's leukemia so he would know I, too, had been the parent of a child prone to develop cancer due to in utero exposure to x-ray.

There is something that has to be said again and again: Not one but many elements have to be taken into consideration when an individual is involved in a biorepair system. There is, unfortunately, a tendency to fragment the healing concept, just as there is a tendency to fragment the disease process. Too many people use the word "wholistic or holistic" in connection with biological therapies without understanding its meaning in the complete sense.

One group feels that psychotherapy is the sole requisite for cancer recovery. Still others put their trust totally in nutrition as the only productive way to deal successfully with diseases like cancer.

Psychic healers, on the other hand, will swear that the laying on of hands will solve all health problems. And, of course, there are yet others who think that herbals, homeopathy or megavitamins represent the major forms of therapy. Any single approach that does not relate to the individual's physiological/psychological need is destined to fail for the vast majority of cancer patients.

Suppose, however, that the patient needs the services of three different disciplines. For example, there may be a biological dysfunction, such as poor thyroid function, poor absorption of nutrients, a circulatory impairment, faulty elimination or any number of problems that cannot be handled by one treatment alone. Each of these breakdowns must be properly diagnosed and corrected. No one form of therapy—even nutrition, supremely important as it is—can help the patient recover when the health problem arises from a different cause.

At a FACT Cancer/Nutrition Convention, Dr. William D. Kelley summed up the difficulties that come with a fragmented view of health. "Yes," he said, "now and then an individual can get well as a result of one of the single-therapy approaches." From his own experience with patients, he could think of a few different therapies from which people came away thinking they had the perfect cure. "But," he added, "each of these individuals had gone to a therapy that just happened to be applicable to their particular health problem, so it worked. But a thousand other people taking that very same path would fail, because it was not adequately suited to their specific health need." If, as is very often the situation, the source of the problem is improper nutrition, and someone prescribed the right dietary regime, it could indeed help that person recover. But very often a well-balanced nutritional program, carefully designed by a practitioner, fails because the biological dysfunction that may be the cause of the breakdown hasn't been corrected.

I might add here that a fragmented approach, with its emphasis on a dramatic "quick fix," has created a dangerous climate where people with little or no training and no clinical experience promote their own favorite therapies. On the basis of their limited experience, they write books and articles, offer resources and advice and enthusiastically advise patients to use a form of treatment or substance that cannot restore health to the organism. This deprives the individual of precious time. People with limited knowledge should be cognizant of the fact that an inexperienced referral to practitioners or institutions about whose work they do not have in-depth knowledge may result in death. An incompetent referral may not include any or all of the services needed by an individual to affect a recovery. The question of what is essential in each particular case is complex. It needs much study and one has to be guided by an experienced practitioner who has competently worked out all the facets of the healing process. Breakdowns which aren't always evident from a superficial examination must be attended to in order to make a biological repair to a body that is producing abnormal cells. Experienced practitioners can make the proper determinations to see that the whole system works harmoniously and, in this way, the patient derives optimum benefit from a program.

Hopefully, in time, the medical community will fill this vacuum of misinformation and provide experienced service for desperate cancer patients. Qualified professionals possessing the background, expertise, training, and diagnostic tools, combined with biological healing directions that have proven their worth, hopefully, will soon give us an unprecedented resource for the restoration of health, including cancer.

We should realize, too, that not every individual can achieve 100% success even with the most sound therapeutic program. There can be a "point of no return" for some. What we can strive for realistically is to attain a state of physical and mental well-being to achieve our optimum life expectancy.

THE WISDOM OF THE BODY

By far, the most important requirement to enable someone to restore one's health and maintain it is to understand physiology (body function). Lack of this understanding makes the individual vulnerable to all sorts of mistakes.

From my experience, it seems obvious that the medical establishment and most of the people doing health research have not had adequate training in physiology. Consequently, evaluations of research projects or physical reactions are skewed. To provide a simple example: when we develop a cough, runny nose, phlegm, diarrhea or similar symptoms that indicate elimination (detoxification) is taking place, the usual treatment is to prescribe an antibiotic or other medicine to alleviate symptoms. If it were recognized that the body had a need to eliminate this unnecessary debris, an antibiotic would not be used to suppress the symptoms. It would be understood that this activity was the wisdom of the body functioning normally, attempting to establish a cleaner and healthier internal environment.

The usual reaction of the medical community—instead of encouraging the body's "housecleaning action"—does the opposite. The use of an antibiotic suppresses the body's attempt to relieve itself of accumulated toxins. If the natural action is suppressed constantly, the body ultimately gives up the effort to eliminate and starts to accumulate. The body is then in the degenerative mode. The body, in its wisdom, constantly fights for survival! It tolerates mistakes because of this innate characteristic.

2. Cancer: The Total Person Approach

If we are what we eat, then Americans are becoming a nation of processed, packaged and preserved people.
—SENATOR ABRAHAM RIBICOFF

From the biological viewpoint, I have tried to show that cancer is a systemic dysfunction resulting from a gradual breakdown of the balance in body chemistry. This breakdown can take place when there is a serious and prolonged disruption of one or more of the body's normal functions, eventually leading to abnormal cell production or degeneration. In this chapter I will provide an overview of the many factors that can contribute to a biological breakdown. Subsequent chapters will go into more depth on individual factors.

The conventional approach, however, holds that cancer is "a type of cell growth that shows some striking differences when compared to normal growth." There are, according to a government publication, over 250 different kinds of cancer. These include, among others, carcinoma, the most common malignant tumor; leukemia, a disease of the blood and bone marrow; lymphoma, a swelling of the lymph glands; and sarcoma, a tumor of certain tissues such as muscle or bone.

In this orthodox definition, cancer is seen as a pathological condition that begins when one or more cells in the body become abnormal. This then triggers an unchecked reproduction which grows into a mass of cells ordinarily called a tumor or blood or bone cancer. If one or more of these cells escapes into another part of the body, and again divides more rapidly than the normal cells, this secondary tumor is referred to as a metastasis.

Unless removed or otherwise corrected, the metastases can spread to other areas of the body. If the disease advances beyond a certain point, it will disrupt the body's biological functioning, destroy or block a vital process and finally cause the death of the organism.

This standard approach to cancer limits the disease, usually, as related to a specific organ or system such as the kidney, breast, skin, blood, liver, lymphatics, pancreas, etc. The invasion of the abnormal cells into other body tissue is attributed to some mysterious compulsion of the original cancer cells to proliferate wildly—for reasons which are theoretical and with which I cannot concur. Scientists don't know if cancer cells continue to grow because the cells receive a signal they no longer understand, or if the signal is actually absent.

Seen in this light, cancer is the tumor itself or the abnormal cells. In contrast to this definition, the biological concept of cancer considers the tumorous cells not to be the cancer, but rather a symptom of the disease. I see cancer as a biochemical breakdown which is provoked by a combination of different causes originating both within and outside the body. It is the end product of a chronic process—that usually begins many years before cancer cells are detected—stemming from a dysfunction in normal body function.

I cannot emphasize strongly enough the implications of this whole-body approach to cancer. Since it suggests that cancer is a biological breakdown, one cannot, therefore, expect to cure cancer by merely removing the tumor, or otherwise treating the site of the tumor only.

Orthodox treatments such as surgery, chemotherapy or radiation may bring about temporary tumor reduction or alleviate symptoms in the patient. But if the breakdown in body chemistry is not corrected, and the system that is producing the cancer cells is not repaired, the cancer, most likely, will return and be considered a metastasis.

In order to rebuild the body's ability to repair itself, enabling it to discontinue the production of abnormal cells, a sound therapeutic program has to consider the entire range of physiological essentials as they apply to each individual. These include as mentioned previously: nutrition, metabolism, detoxification, correcting body misalignment including the temporomandibular joint (TMJ), stress control, improving glandular function and correcting any physiological dysfunction. Where indicated, various nontoxic therapies such as botanicals, fever therapy (hyperthermia), immunotherapy, and cellular therapy, may be of added help but should not be considered the primary treatment. Chapter 9 will explain these therapies in depth.

Because cancer is the culmination of different offenses to the body that have occurred over a long period of time, the restoration of health is never a quick or easy process. Almost always, it will take a number of years to bring about the full repair needed to achieve optimal health restoration—often with healing inflammations. The patient's cooperation is necessary to eliminate the lifestyle abuses and mistakes that have contributed to the disease. Unfortunately, sometimes the breakdown has gone too far to be repaired by any means. This is usually the *exception*, not the more common occurrence.

WHAT ARE THE CAUSES OF CANCER?

If scientists knew the answer, you probably wouldn't be reading this book; there would be no need to continue raising research funds, because they would know how to prevent and cure this most dreaded disease.

Different theories on what causes cancer continue to be advanced in orthodox circles. A while back, for example, there was much discussion about the role viruses played in relation to cancer, but no concrete scientific evidence has verified the theory. Some clinical evidence suggests that different forms of cancer could be attributed to various substances in the diet—such as fat, coffee, sugar substitutes, red dye, etc. It should be noted that these theories very often arouse controversy and disagreements among doctors, scientists and institutions dealing with cancer.

In recent years there has been general agreement that a number of toxic materials, known as carcinogens, are cancer-causing. These substances include chemicals such as asbestos, coal tar, vinyl chloride, and others, which may be found in small quantities in the air, water, food, home and the workplace. Other factors that are now commonly accepted as cancer-causing include excessive x-rays and smoking. The latest concept the medical community is hoping will be the answer is the gene theory—the theoretical assignment of certain diseases and characteristics to specific genes. This is still unproven and may become another illusory direction.

At a nutrition seminar sponsored by the American Cancer Society during the 1970s, one presenter delivered a talk which included many concepts which we at FACT have held from our very origins. The discussion of possible cancer causes included drugs, stress, radiation, pollution, additives in food, diet, etc. I found this movement toward the biological viewpoint of cancer very heartening and can only applaud many of the things that are taking place in the medical profession today that would have seemed impossible just a few years ago. There are signs that many in the medical community are moving closer to accepting FACT's idea that a physiological impairment (biological breakdown) is the vital factor in the formation of abnormal cells; however, there is still no official acceptance.

The Precipitating Factors

In the previous chapter, I discussed the various ways in which different kinds of systemic dysfunctions in life processes can lead to a biological breakdown. At this point, however, you might wonder: What are the factors that may cause this biological breakdown—and why do these factors end with disease in one individual and not in another?

There are a number of harmful elements—a weak constitution, chronic stress, dangerous chemicals in the air, water or workplace—which can in some situations provoke a biological breakdown in an individual who is already vulnerable because of the above conditions.

I can give you the example of my own daughter, Arlene, who died of leukemia. I was x-rayed just before she was born because it was discovered she was breached (the feet were engaged in the birth canal instead of the head). After she died, my husband and I found many instances where it was claimed that x-ray to the fetus harms the baby's gonads and can produce leukemia. We even learned that x-ray of the reproductive area prior to conception can produce leukemia in the offspring. This is due to the fact that eggs available for fertilization are affected by the x-ray. Some children can survive for years and possibly fulfill their life cycle; others may die at an earlier age than Arlene. Arlene became a leukemia victim at the age of twenty-nine. When a person who is vulnerable to disease is subjected to harmful conditions such as excessive x-rays, stress, drugs, and carcinogenic additives in food, these precipitating factors can trigger a breakdown in body chemistry. The precipitating factor is not ordinarily the direct cause of the disease. Where there is already vulnerability or susceptibility to disease, it can be the final insult to the vulnerable body.

The Carcinogenic Component

The World Health Organization has estimated that between 75% to 80% of all cancers are "environmentally induced." A book, *Toxic Deception: How the Chemical Industry Manipulates Science, Bends the Law, and Endangers Your Health,* by Dan Fagin, Marianne Lavelle and the Center for Public Integrity (Monroe: Common Courage Press, 1999), claims that over "70,000 man-made chemicals are being sold today. About 300 have been identified as cancer-causing agents in animal tests by the National Toxicology Program (NTP) researchers. The true number of carcinogenic chemicals is probably far higher, since the program has not conducted even preliminary screenings on more than 80 percent of the chemicals currently on the market."

Occupational carcinogens are, of course, a serious problem, affecting millions of working Americans. But carcinogens can also do their damage as environmental hazards outside the factories in the form of smog, smoke, dust, coal tar, oils, polluted water, and so forth. So it's not just the chemical carcinogens that should concern us, but the accumulation and interaction of the incredible number of man-made toxic materials that don't belong in the human environment. It will never be possible to protect ourselves from *all carcinogens, ergo, it is essential that we develop and maintain strong host resistance.*

It is important to remember that being exposed to a chemical carcinogen does not necessarily by itself cause cancer. Otherwise, all of the people exposed to a cancer-causing chemical in one particular workplace would get the disease. In actuality, only a small percentage do. As we have already seen, other destructive factors are usually present in the individual, and, of course, no two people have the same constitution or the same degree of susceptibility.

Exposure to carcinogens is inescapable; they exist wherever we turn— chemical cleaning supplies in our homes, the stores we shop, the streets, our cars and subways, even when we are on vacation far away from the crowded, dirty cities. We breathe them in the air as smoke, carbon dioxide, nitrogen oxide, gasoline fumes and a whole mix of other pollutants. We find them in our tap water as fluoride, chlorine and other harmful residues. They show up in our fresh fruits and vegetables as residues of pesticides, chemical fertilizers, and weed killers. They adulterate our foodstuffs as additives, preservatives, coloring agents, sweeteners and countless other chemical offenses. They follow us into our homes as aerosols, insecticides, benzene products and deodorants.

No one knows for certain exactly how much exposure to a carcinogen—or for that matter to any dangerous substance—it takes to finally break down the resistance to cancer. I am certain, however, that there is *no such thing as safe exposure to any cancer-causing material.* Only host resistance protects us from harm. Even limited exposure to toxic substances, in an individual who already has other weaknesses, can lead to cancer either in a short time or as much as 20 or 30 years. This latent period is the time it takes for the outward manifestation of the disease.

In addition, the damage brought about by exposure to toxic chemicals is usually cumulative, so that the more exposure, the greater the damage. Research studies have also shown that combinations of chemicals, acting together on a human being, will produce a more explosive reaction in a shorter period of time than any single chemical.

Nature never intended for the human organism to handle such a large number of chemical substances with which our bodies are bombarded. We need to maintain a competent defense system to withstand the onslaught and avoid, as much as possible, the offensive conditions. Temporarily, the body will use its resources to eliminate the toxins. Eventually, however, the vulnerable individual who is subjected to the constant barrage, in violation of Nature's requirements, will be unable to eliminate the accumulated toxins. This is because the elimination mechanism becomes overloaded and exhausted. The end result could be cancer or other degenerative diseases.

The Effect of Drugs

What I have said about carcinogens and other harmful chemicals also applies to many pharmaceuticals which inundate our drug stores and constitute a major form of conventional treatment. Like all other non-biological materials, many drugs also have harmful properties which cannot necessarily be evaluated until after many years of use. The pharmaceutical industry is required by the Food and Drug Administration (FDA) to test drugs on experimental animals and to have human trials before being approved as safe. Enough time is not always factored into the conclusions nor are animal systems equivalent to those of humans. In most instances only one drug is used at a time, whereas a person may be using a variety of medicines and be exposed to other environmental factors simultaneously. It is impossible to know with certainty whether a drug that has won approval by the FDA is not carcinogenic when it acts in combination with other drugs.

The list of drugs—prescribed or bought over-the-counter—is simply staggering. It includes everything from sleeping pills to birth control pills; from tension medications to antibiotics; from analgesics to cough syrups; headache medications to gas relievers. Buying and relying on pharmaceuticals is an American obsession. It has made the pharmaceutical industry one of the richest in our nation. We rarely tolerate discomfort if there is a substance to provide immediate relief. It is rare, indeed, for people to think that healing is possible without medication.

I would not presume to advise any of my readers whether or not to use any particular drug. That is a decision only you and your doctor can make. What I can do is provide the kind of information that will help individuals participate intelligently as medical consumers.

In this regard, I can only repeat what I have said before about any substance which is produced chemically. Even if it is not carcinogenic in the official sense, cumulative effects are uncertain. Although drugs have a place in health care, if used indiscriminately—as far too many people do—they can create serious health problems. One must always weigh the risks against the so-called benefits. A drug may temporarily relieve a painful symptom, but in terms of comparing its immediate and long-term effects, is the drug actually worth it?

As far as drugs and medications are concerned, the pharmaceutical industry is no longer using the safer botanicals that were used in the past. In fact, you will find fewer and fewer botanicals listed in the pharmacopoeia despite the fact that they do not cause many of the dangerous complications that can be caused by the drugs in use today. (Note: The first edition of the *Physician's Desk Reference (PDR) for Herbal Medicines* was published in the year 2000).*

If you've had an opportunity to examine the side-effect information caused by drugs, which is usually available in the PDR,* you would find the listing quite terrifying. FACT sometimes publishes the adverse reactions to a drug in *Cancer Forum*, the official FACT publication; reading these reac-

---

*PDR (Physician's Desk Reference) is a book used by professionals to acquire detailed information about all the drugs manufactured by the pharmaceutical industry.

tions is a sobering experience. They range from severe skin rashes and hearing disturbances, through intestinal ulcerations and hemorrhage, toxic hepatitis to aplastic anemia, and in some instances actual fatalities. Pharmaceutical companies claim that these are unusual and infrequent reactions, but the fact remains that there is no telling what dangerous effects the drugs can have on a person.

Most of these drugs simply alleviate symptoms; they do not contain curative elements. If a drug is for coughing, all it can do is prevent the cough reflex and halt the flow of mucous and other wastes that *should* be eliminated from the body. The function of diuretics is to help stimulate the flow of water from the body. The action of drugs is entirely different from those of nutrients or botanicals which can focus on causes and, in this way, help the system make the biorepairs necessary to overcome a breakdown and its symptoms. Pharmaceuticals have a place in the health market; they are useful in a crisis. Unfortunately, they are used too indiscriminately and casually.

Smoke at Your Own Risk

I don't think it's necessary to belabor the hazardous effects of smoking. Just about every adult and teenager in the United States should be aware of the danger when a major cigarette company admits publicly, and media attention is focused on, the carcinogenicity of smoking. There is ample evidence that the startlingly high rate of cancer of the lungs, larynx, esophagus, throat and mouth is largely attributable to smoking. And a recent study claims it also causes colon cancer.

The evidence is no longer disputed that tobacco tar, nicotine and other chemical by-products which are released in smoking are detrimental to the lung mucosa, arteries and air sacs. They also cut down on oxygen intake, and increase the risk of high-blood pressure, heart disease and other circulatory ailments.

Excessive X-rays & Radiation

There is, of course, complete agreement that overexposure to x-rays and other forms of radiation can increase the incidence of cancer. The disagreement among scientists and physicians is: just how much radiation can be considered safe?

In diagnosis and therapy, it is always better to rely on diagnostic techniques which avoid x-rays. There are times, however, when x-rays are essential. Even when they are appropriate, it is important to exercise caution by selecting a laboratory with modern equipment that uses low-dose radiation and limits the number of x-rays to no more than what is absolutely necessary.

Too often, x-rays are prescribed without sufficient consideration of the x-ray history of the patient, or whether or not x-rays are absolutely necessary. Some time ago, the Food and Drug Administration (FDA) recognized this by issuing guidelines to the effect that people should keep their own record of the amount of x-rays to which they are exposed.

Although there is no exact method known for measuring what would be a safe allowance, 40 rems are considered tolerable by the FDA for an individual's entire lifetime. A diagnostic evaluation of the thyroid, which includes radioactive isotopes, uses up a 24-year allowance!

When an x-ray is indicated, for whatever purpose, it's up to the patient to ask the doctor or radiologist just what the potency of the x-ray is. The doctor and you can make an informed decision based on this knowledge as to how few x-rays are necessary.

Sunlight is a form of natural radiation that is essential to good health. No therapeutic program would be complete without its healing effects. People, like plants, need the sun's warming rays for nourishment, energy, relaxation and to help build and repair the tissues and bone. However, overdoing exposure to the sun's rays can have as negative an effect as x-rays.

Mind/Body Connection

Attention should be paid to the effect of stress on the body as well as mind—and on its relation to *disease and immunity*. Our best authority on this subject is Hans Selye, M.D., who conducted stress research for many years at the University of Montreal. It is also worth calling your attention to Walter B. Cannon, M.D., a world-renowned physician-researcher who was head of the physiology research department at Harvard University during the 1920s and 30s. He was one of the originators of the concept that hyperactivity of our organs and hormonal imbalance can cause diseases which are clearly related to nervous stimuli such as physical disorders, and ultimately organ damage and destruction.

Dr. Cannon called the body's reaction to stress "the flight or fight" response. It is this automatic reaction which enables our bodies to defend themselves or to flee when necessary for self preservation. Whenever this reaction occurs, our stress hormones from the adrenal glands and from our own neural activity are secreted rapidly, making this emergency response possible. As part of this reaction, muscle tension is increased, heart rate and blood pressure rise, the pupils dilate, perspiration increases, etc. Normally, when the danger passes, the body regains its balance from this agitated condition—heartbeat and blood pressure fall, muscle tension relaxes and respiration normalizes.

This emergency response to danger is one that has been instinctual for millions of years. Today, however, we are assaulted constantly with personal tensions, social pressures and other stress-inducing factors. Some of us can cope well with these pressures. Other individuals, however, cannot deal with this *chronic* stress. It reaches a point where it can exhaust their bodies and eventually, if unchecked, seriously upset the biological balance. The result can be a biological breakdown as varied as high blood pressure, heart attacks—or in combination with other factors—degenerative diseases such as cancer.

Dr. Selye has fully documented the ways in which stress—as a result of the continuing pattern of overstimulation—wreaks havoc on the endocrine system. If the individual can't handle this stress physically or mentally, the organs are not going to produce the proper secretions, thus upsetting the body's ability to perform normally. This disruption in the nerve system can also interfere with competent waste elimination. It can prevent the lungs from functioning properly, so that not enough oxygen is supplied to the bloodstream and not enough waste is expelled. It can interfere with normal food metabolism and circulation of nutrients to the cells for normal cell production.

Let me give you a more specific example: You may know that the vagus nerve, located where the esophagus connects with the stomach, triggers the secretion of hydrochloric acid (an essential digestive component) into the stomach. When we are under severe stress, there may be an enormous oversecretion of this digestive juice, eventually causing the development of an ulcer. If stress is allowed to go on too long without regulation, it can produce a chronic condition. Keith Sedlacek, M.D., a well-known authority on biofeedback for stress control, has cited evidence that some cases of cancer are related to chronic stress, and an increase in *chronic stress lowers resistance to cancer growth.*

Following is a quote from Dr. Sedlacek's book, *How to Avoid Stress Before*

It Kills You, "Clearly, your attitude toward life, your mood (optimistic or pessimistic), helps create the atmosphere that assists your defense system in repairing small wounds, bruises, and infections. This system also tries to destroy strange cells, such as those of cancer."

Stress, as Dr. Sedlacek points out, is a normal component of life. When you are in a reasonably healthy state, your body will be able to minimize the effects of stress by integrating it into your life. If you are already in ill health, tensions can add to the burden, so that the body may suffer a serious disruption of normal functioning.

Lifestyle Abuses

Nature designed the body to work harmoniously, and for humans to live long, healthy lives. The body is equipped with all kinds of self-regulatory processes to carry out metabolism, maintain a sound biological balance in all of its functions, and repair the damages that arise in the course of normal, everyday living. But you cannot *constantly* violate Nature's requirements. As wonderful as your body is, it needs sufficient rest to recuperate its healing abilities. If you continue to subject your body to excessive behavior, abuse and neglect, sooner or later the result will be a breakdown in some *vital life process.*

If, for example, your body requires sleep, fighting it violates one of life's essentials. Sleep deprivation can produce all sorts of health complications. I knew a man who wouldn't allow himself to sleep for more than four hours nightly, because he wanted to utilize all the time he could for learning. After doing this for many years, he developed cancer. It's possible his body rebelled due to weakened host resistance as a result of lack of sleep. One cannot continuously violate Nature's laws without suffering consequences.

The same can be said for constantly violating any of Nature's requirements: poor eating habits, overeating or undereating; inadequate elimination of wastes, unnecessary high-risk behavior, and letting negative emotions *rule your life.*

Most people who choose biological therapies readily understand the need to improve their diets, to utilize supplements only as they are indicated for the individual, or to find effective means of eliminating their body wastes. It is not easy to recognize and change emotional patterns of lifetime abuses that have become so ingrained as to seem "normal." I am thinking, in particular, of one cancer patient who followed a biologically-sound diet, took enzymes and other essential nutrients faithfully, detoxi-fied when her practitioner suggested this, and was extremely careful to rid her body of wastes daily. In short, she was the "perfect" patient, and yet there was little or no improvement in her health.

Conversations with this woman revealed that she was a professional writer who was concerned with her work to the point of obsession. Com-petitive and compulsive, she would sit hunched over her typewriter for many hours at a stretch, her muscles tense, her breathing impaired, hard-ly aware of what was going on around her. Despite her doctor's warnings, she denied herself real vacations, regular periods of relaxation and exer-cise, and a space for calm and contemplation. Is it any wonder that her body continued to show outward manifestations of biological impair-ment—indigestion, rapid heartbeat, cold hands and feet, acid/alkaline imbalance, and so forth? It was evident to me that, unless she broke the vicious cycle of overwork, there might be no way she could overcome the severe biological breakdown that had caused her illness in the first place. If one wants to use that much abused word "wholistic," this woman is an excellent example of the profound interrelationship between the way we think and feel, the way we live, and the way our bodies function.

Spinal Misalignment

Unlike the above precipitating factors, spinal misalignment is a structural impairment within the body itself. This form of structural imbalance, howev-er, is important and too often disregarded in evaluating a patient's condition.

When misalignment occurs, pressure is exerted on the sensitive nerve ends located between the vertebrae. This depresses the nerve's ability to relay strong normal signals to the target organs, which in turn interrupts the flow of messages from the brain to the organs. In some instances, spinal misalignment may cause distressing physical symptoms as well—pain, spasm, inflammation and contractions. The chart on pages 142–143 shows how the various nerve ends located between the vertebrae of the spine connect directly with specific organs. These include organs whose functions are triggered by the autonomic nerve system—heart, lungs, liver, colon, endocrine system, etc.

In order to maintain health, this involuntary nerve system has to work harmoniously and as efficiently as possible. When the spine is aligned, signals originating in the brain are transferred unimpeded to the nerve ends, making it possible for the organs receiving the signals to respond normally. However, when the spine alignment is distorted—for whatever reason—one or more nerves may tend to be pinched or blocked. The pressure at the nerve end, caused by this faulty alignment, will prevent the related organ from performing its work adequately.

If you study the chart of the nerve system, you can see for yourself the wide range of abnormal conditions that can follow from pressure on, or interference with, these nerves. These ailments include, to mention only a few: poor bowel or kidney elimination, inadequate oxygen intake, improper digestion, sluggish circulation, bladder trouble, etc. At a certain stage, in combination with other damaging factors, the misalignment can produce a general weakening or even breakdown of an organ system that can progress from compromised host resistance to chronic or degenerative disease.

Because spinal misalignment can cause so many symptomatic and underlying health problems, practitioners may advise the patient to see a skilled osteopath or chiropractor to make the necessary adjustments to correct the spinal condition and free the nerve system of interference.

Temporomandibular Joint (TMJ) Disorder

Still another form of physical impairment that too often goes unnoticed is caused by a displacement of the temporomandibular joint (TMJ). When this joint is out of alignment, the resulting jaw stress can create numerous multiple symptoms that appear in the head, neck and eyes.

What causes the TMJ maladjustment? It can be the result of any unnatural strain on the lower jaw and teeth. It may also be caused by extractions, dental alterations, grinding one's teeth, or by an injury to the chin or head that changes the position of the jaw joint.

Repositioning of the joint is usually done by dentists who specialize in TMJ adjustments. For further information, please see my discussion of the temporomandibular joint in Chapter 8.

Inadequate Oxygen

The act of breathing seems to be such an automatic function; consequently people ignore the important role oxygen plays in maintaining good health—or, conversely, in contributing to bad health.

We know that it is the job of the lungs to bring oxygen into the blood-stream and to expel carbon dioxide and other waste products. If we breathe too shallowly—because of tension, poor posture, spinal misalignment or for other reasons—we will be unable to take in enough oxygen to eliminate waste adequately.

Shallow breathing can, in combination with other negative factors, lead to a loss of vitality and cause fatigue, tension, headaches, circulatory ailments, as well as other physical problems. It is important to realize the fact that oxygen deprivation can have a potent effect on the health of the whole body.

Lack of Exercise

Like inadequate breathing, the lack of exercise or other forms of physical activity can be responsible, in no small measure, for a wide variety of health problems. Sedentary living, for example, can create sluggish circu-lation in the lymphatic and circulatory systems, thereby decreasing the supply of oxygen and nutrients to the cells, and impairing the drainage of toxic wastes. Everyone can exercise providing it is limited to their individ-ual physical tolerance and not done to the point of exhaustion.

It is interesting to compare our own advanced societies with those of so-called primitive peoples who were so much more physically vigorous than we are. A well-documented research study contrasted the nomadic Eskimos of old with their modern counterparts. The former fished, worked and moved constantly, while Eskimos today work at sedentary jobs, eat canned-food products for easy living and have abandoned a life of natural activity. In little more than a generation, heart disease, diabetes and degenerative diseases such as cancer have shown up at an alarming rate. Can anyone doubt that this combination of chronic physical inactivity, improper dietary habits and other ills of civilization have harmed the bodies and minds of people who were once so fit? I think the lesson of this research study is clear for all of us to learn: when we neglect exercising our body's muscles and organs, we are at great risk of impairing our well-being.

Poor Nutrition

Increasingly, it is being recognized that faulty nutrition is one of the most important causative elements in the biological breakdown process. There now exists an impressive and growing bibliography of research studies which correlate nutrition with diseases such as arthritis, heart trouble and cancer itself. Cancer has been specifically linked with nutritional excesses, deficiencies and imbalances. Periodically, conventional scientists, physicians and government health agencies issue public statements to the effect that a nutritional item can play a vital role in protecting against cancer.

I don't want to leave the impression that nutritional concepts which we at FACT support have won broad acceptance in orthodox circles. There's still work to do. Unfortunately, we still live at a time when doctors have not been taught nutrition as an integral part of the overall medical curriculum. They've been trained to treat symptoms after they have developed, but know little about nutrition to prevent disease and maintain health. There is not yet—so far as I know—a traditional public or private hospital that fully incorporates what I consider to be a sound nutritional program as part of its treatment regime for cancer or other degenerative diseases.

Exactly what is meant when we say that a particular nutritional regime is unwholesome or unbalanced? To begin with, it means that an individual is just not getting all of the nutritional components required to produce healthy cells and maintain the integrity of the body. The human body requires only minute quantities of each nutrient, but every one of these substances is essential for healthy cell production and repair. Among the many substances which the body needs are: proteins, carbohydrates, fatty acids, glucose, sodium, vitamins, minerals, trace minerals, enzymes and, of course water.

These substances—primarily obtained from food sources—are needed to nourish, repair and produce healthy cells. And all of the food elements need to be metabolized competently to achieve the ultimate goal of good health. When one or more of these nutrients are missing consistently from our diets, the body has a way of compensating by using stored elements from muscles, bones, nails and teeth in order to maintain homeostasis. This is fortunate for all of us in that the human system can sustain life for a long time despite a lot of abuse—nutritional or otherwise. It is unfortunate, however, in that it cannot be determined easily when the abuse has reached the point that is no longer tolerable. The neglect will result in a biological breakdown which is the beginning of disease.

Some of the breakdowns are obvious and well-known. For example, if you do not supply the body with enough vitamin C, scurvy can develop. If there is not enough vitamin B in the diet, you may develop beriberi. If you do not consume enough protein, the result will be loss of muscle tone or hair. A lack of calcium will manifest in osteoporosis. A tremendous amount of research has been done to determine what will happen when one or another nutrient is missing from our food supply. No one doubts that when a deficiency is long-lasting, and is constant, it may lead to a symptomatic manifestation of a problem.

The question as to when, and under what circumstances, poor nutrition can trigger a degenerative disease like cancer is complex and thorny. Likely, chronic and extreme nutritional deficiencies and abuses, in conjunction with an individual's constitution, state of health, mental attitude, and pattern of waste elimination will contribute to the process. What we do know is: every person has a different tolerance to nutritional deficiency, as well as a different level of immunological defense against disease. At some point, however, if pushed too far, the human system will no longer be able to protect itself from a biological breakdown. One has only to look at the frightening cancer statistics in the United States to know that this is true.

Faulty Elimination

Our body has four main avenues of waste elimination—colon, kidneys, lungs and skin. Elimination of body wastes is as crucial to the restoration and maintenance of health as the intake of our nutritional fuel. At times, it can be even more imperative. This is not the usual stance of the medical profession. As a matter of fact, this issue tends to be controversial. The research done by Dr. Alexis Carrel at Rockefeller University (keeping chicken heart cells alive in a petri dish by providing correct nourishment and daily waste removal) and the papers presented by Sir William Arbuthnot Lane, M.D., on his broad experience restoring health by encouraging colon cleanliness, validates the importance of maintaining a clean colon and healthy musculature. When toxins accumulate to the point where they cannot be properly eliminated, the cells and lymphatics store the waste temporarily and continuously recirculate it in the bloodstream in the body's attempt at elimination.

The source of these accumulated toxins can be undigested food, polluted water and air, drugs, dangerous chemical by-products, bacterial wastes, and sloughed off cells. Stress, too, can be responsible for upsetting the metabolism and interfering with the body's ability to rid itself of waste products. Skeletal misalignment, which weakens signals to the organs of elimination such as the liver, kidneys and the bowels is another complication that needs to be addressed.

Whatever the reason may be for the accumulation of body wastes, it can reach a concentration that completely overtaxes the system of elimination. Unless measures are then taken to detoxify the system, the patient's efforts to restore health will be frustrated.

As Sir William Arbuthnot Lane, M.D.; J. H. Tilden, M.D.; J. Harvey Kellogg, M.D. and others have shown, the colon, the primary organ of elimination, is the key to the maintenance of overall health. When our diet is wrong, or when there is chronic indigestion or sluggish colon musculature, thus interfering with full elimination, pockets of hard, plaster-like waste may form on the colon wall and remain there. Or else, because of the type of food eaten, the transit time of the food moving through the colon may be too long. In any event, while dawdling through the bowel, the harbored toxic putrefaction may be absorbed by the body by means of the portal vein. These toxins are absorbed into the bloodstream and possibly stored in the cells or lymphatics.

Of course, other organs are part of this elimination process as well. If the liver is not cleansing the bloodstream adequately or if the kidneys are not functioning well, these organs will be unable to properly filter out the harmful chemicals. If the lungs don't expel sufficient waste products of cell metabolism, and the skin doesn't throw off other wastes by means of perspiration, the retained toxins will be stored by the cells and tissues. Waste may then accumulate beyond the body's ability to eliminate adequately until it becomes a destructive source of disease for the entire body.

Some additional substances that can add to an overload of waste in the cells are food additives, preservatives, drugs, fluoride or chlorine in the water, chemicals in household cleaners, cosmetics, x-rays, and microwaves. Consider, for example, the chemicals, synthetics, coloring agents, pesticide residues, antibiotics, hormones, bleaches, emulsifiers, artificial sweeteners, tenderizers and other alien substances that are to be found in the shopping cart of an average American. Does anyone have any idea of the tens of billions of dollars that are spent annually on useless calories of junk foods—everything from hot dogs, through candy bars to soda pop? Or on white flour, white rice or refined sugar whose natural nutrients have been processed out of existence? Or the foods that have been pickled, canned, bottled and preserved into a state equivalent to embalming?

When any chemicalized food or, in fact, any toxin is taken into the body in the minute amounts that are cumulative, the resulting buildup can be specifically injurious to normal body function. The body will use its resources to eliminate the toxins. As long as the body can keep pace with the strain that is imposed on it as a result of accumulated toxins, it can avert a major biological breakdown. The body may divert the toxins to the lung in an effort to eliminate them; this may surface as a cold, runny nose, mucus, sore throat, or sneezing. Symptoms of the overload may also manifest as fever, chronic headache, gastrointestinal problems, exhaustion, depression, sallow skin, rashes, nausea, diarrhea or other relatively minor problems.

Each individual has a different capacity for getting rid of toxins. That is why one person can eat all sorts of foods containing chemicals and still process them down to complete elimination, while others eating the same foods will develop a backup causing a storage of wastes. By and large, however, the elimination system is able to do a remarkable job in ridding the body of toxic substances that are the by-products of chemicalized foods and putrefaction. We all know people who are relatively healthy in spite of the fact that they break every conceivable rule of sound nutrition. The comment by Nobel prize winner Dr. Albert Szent Gyorgyi very much pertains to this point: "When I see what people eat, I am not very astonished when they get sick; I'm extremely surprised that they survive."

I feel obliged to present all of the negative forces—so many avoidable—that can impinge on one's health. It may be frightening to the reader. It is not meant to be. The reason for listing the whole range of hazards is just to be sure that one recognizes them so steps can be taken before they develop into a pathology. Nature has indeed endowed us with an extraordinary capacity to tolerate abuses. With knowledge we can avoid challenging her to excess.

3. Repairing the Biological Breakdown

The will to live is not a theoretical abstraction,
but a physiologic reality with therapeutic characteristics.
—NORMAN COUSINS

I n my experience with cancer patients, I have observed that there is no "quick fix" in bringing this illness under control. The biological breakdown which opens the door to cancer is in itself the end product of many and complex precipitating causes. The damage which the body suffers as a consequence of this long-term degenerative process often can be quite extensive. Almost always, the biological therapies that are used to help the body repair the dysfunctions will require a considerable length of time and will seldom be without highs and lows of energy as the body uses vitality for healing. Therefore, when the body is in the healing phase, energy is diverted from daily activity, signalling it is time to rest. Invariably, cancer is a problem that has taken years—even decades—to develop. It needs time and patience to repair.

I have seen that standard treatments for cancer have by and large proved ineffective for long-term recovery. This is evident, not only from the grim cancer statistics, but from the growing realization on the part of many in the medical community that radiation, surgery and chemotherapy are not the real solution to the problem. In fact increasingly people in the medical profession realize that some of these therapies in and of themselves can often prove harmful to the patients.

Dr. John Bailar, III, a Harvard statistician, reviewed cancer statistics covering a twenty year period of survival, disregarding the artificial five-year-survival yardstick. The investigation concluded that the death rate per 100,000 had increased despite the fact that the five-year-survival marker seemed to leave the impression that cancer treatment over all had improved.

There is a mistaken assumption among doctors and patients that the mere reduction of a tumor mass represents a cancer cure. The focus of current cancer research is, and has been, tumor destruction. To date, this approach has not been the solution nor does the medical establishment claim that it has the cure for cancer. The term "cure" refers only to a five-year survival period; even that is not achieved in all forms of cancer. Obviously, getting rid of the tumorous mass, whether it is done with surgery, radiation, toxic substances (chemotherapy) or hormone inhibitors, is not the answer. Since these procedures do nothing to correct the cause of abnormal cell production, they can merely buy time.

ALTERNATIVE CLAIMS

I am terribly troubled by the lack of understanding that people have when they are searching for a therapy outside of radiation and chemotherapy; that is, when they are looking for an "alternative" therapy. Unless the therapy is biologically sound, it is not truly an alternative; it is just a variation of the present system. Some of the so-called alternatives can be just as toxic as chemotherapy. I am also troubled by the exaggerated claims of success that are being made for many so-called alternative therapies. Some of them are beneficial or produce meager results, others have not been used long enough to evaluate properly, or are ineffective for long-term recovery. Yet many unskilled people are promoting therapies to cancer patients who are in life-threatening situations, are "grabbing at straws" and afraid to ignore any suggestion for fear it will be the one to perform the miracle they are seeking.

Kathie Keaton, the wife of the publisher of *Penthouse Magazine*, appeared on television leaving the impression that she was cured of cancer by using hydrazine sulfate. Although hydrazine sulfate is a chemotherapy, it can be classified as an alternative only because it has not been accepted by the FDA. Sadly, it violates the precept of a biologically-sound system. The flood of calls at the FACT office due to Kathie Keaton's media appearance was overwhelming. Callers never waited to see if her recovery sustained. The nature of cancer is such that one can often survive with treatment, without treatment, with minimal treatment, or different kinds of treatment, for possibly as long as four to six years or even longer, before the body runs into serious difficulty. Sometimes the survival time depends on the particular form of cancer, or the constitution of the patient or the level of host resistance. To attribute the success of any particular therapy without patiently waiting for a sufficient number of years is extremely incompetent. And to assume that one person's success with a program makes it a viable method for all is no less incompetent. There are no miracles or instant solutions—and that goes for the gamut of alternatives as well as conventional treatments.

Calling an alternative substance an alternative treatment is confusing. FACT's conception of an alternative therapy has always been a wholistic system of applying all of the needed components for host repair. Using an alternative product is not my criterion for a good cancer therapy. A system that focuses on healthy cell production is a real alternative and more productive than one that focuses on cancer cell destruction. When we used the term "alternative" in our original title, the *Foundation for Alternative Cancer Therapies* (FACT); it represented a biologically-sound, comprehensive system.

People can find a great deal of information on alternative procedures or techniques that promise an effortless answer to a pathology that was brought on by a lifetime of health-denying behavior or other damaging factors. The cancer patient may then think that all that's needed is to get the magic potion, the proper injections, do as the doctor orders, and they are well on their way to real recovery. I can evaluate every therapy and come to the same conclusion—there is no miracle, whether it is a botanical, a fever treatment, a form of immunotherapy, a stress-control system, psychotherapy, or cell therapy. I am not minimizing the value of any of these treatments as adjunctives. But again, I must say, *if it doesn't correct the breakdown in body chemistry, which is the bedrock of cell production, it is going to provide limited or unpredictable value.*

This point has been difficult to get across to patients, doctors, and others who lack an understanding of the physiology of the biological healing process. People who are writing dramatic stories about cancer cures achieved with so-called alternatives need to understand this point. I can appreciate that many are doing it out of sympathy for the patient. Nevertheless, without proper information, training, or clinical experience, grievous errors can be made.

Just because individuals have nutritional knowledge or use buzzwords like "detoxification" or "immunity" it does not automatically validate their qualifications to correct a biological dysfunction. What is necessary is the experience and ability to successfully evaluate and integrate the multi-aspects of the biological approach so that the body as a whole will be *restored to normal function.*

CONVENTIONAL THERAPIES

As discussed before, conventional medicine continues primarily to depend on surgery, radiation and chemotherapy as its major therapeutic tools. Because these are so widely publicized, and so little understood by the general public, I should like to comment more fully on each of these treatments for cancer.

Surgical intervention consists of excising the tumor from the affected part of the body whenever possible. Though it is an orthodox treatment, it is biologically less offensive to the integrity of the body than radiation, chemotherapy or hormone inhibitors. Surgery can debulk the cancer mass but needs to be considered carefully as there are some types of surgery, such as bypasses, that violate the integrity of the body and make normal restoration impossible. Unfortunately, sometimes surgery is imperative in order to relieve the body if the condition is life-threatening.

A bleak report prepared several decades ago by the National Cancer Institute stated that the various surgical approaches did not seem to have made a great difference in the outcome of a large number of gastric and kidney cancer patients. The unfortunate reality is that these conclusions are still valid today.

Chemotherapy is a treatment that invades the whole system. The toxic chemicals travel through the veins or are taken orally, so they are distributed throughout the body—exposing normal as well as cancer cells to the poisons. Chemotherapy is used on the principle that one or more of these numerous drugs will destroy cancer cells before destroying the patient. Sometimes the opposite happens. I am personally familiar with two cases when chemotherapy, not the cancer, caused the death of the patient.

A government booklet, entitled *Cancer Treatment,* states that the chemicals themselves are capable of causing cancer: "Since the drugs strike at the heart of genetic material, they can cause aberrations which may cause second cancers if normal cells are affected." The same booklet warns that anticancer drugs can "make people feel very uncomfortable with nausea, vomiting and diarrhea." They also tend to depress the production of blood cells in the bone marrow resulting in a decrease in blood counts.

There is a risk of serious problems, such as leukemia, bleeding, uncontrollable infections and anemia. Some drugs used for this purpose have also been known to damage the function of the kidneys, heart, liver or immune system.

Periodically a new chemotherapy is announced with great fanfare as being more effective and less harmful than others. After a while it is succeeded by still another drug with even greater claims. But I believe that subjecting a sick system to toxic substances, except temporarily in a crisis, is not a logical way of treating cancer. Here again, there is nothing in the chemotherapy *to repair the systemic breakdown that is responsible for the production of abnormal cells.*

Radiation, the third conventional treatment, consists of bombarding the body with therapeutic doses of x-rays as a means of killing cancer cells and thus shrinking the tumor mass. Although it is a local form of treatment, it kills normal cells as well as cancer cells. In actuality, however, even with the newest megavoltage or pinpointed instruments, radiation also affects normal internal tissues.

Arguments as to whether these three forms of orthodox therapy do indeed improve the cancer cure rate are complex and contradictory. Haydn Bush, M.D., former Director of the London Regional Cancer Centre in Canada, states "Despite claims to the contrary, treatment today offers little more hope than it did a generation ago. The results have shown little survival advantage for any treatment." Reduction of mortality in different forms of cancer, as a result of the use of anticancer drugs or radiation, shows little clinical evidence that real recovery has been achieved. In any event, both chemotherapy and radiation violate the integrity of the body, and subject an already weakened body to damage that can only hinder genuine biological repair.

Ultimately, I hope the medical community, after debulking the tumor, adopts as its *first choice of treatment* a system to effect a biorepair before incurring irreparable damage with radiation or chemotherapy, or creating hormonal imbalance with hormone inhibitors. And that oncologists would only resort to the system of buying time if the body fails to respond due to the advanced stage of the disease or because the breakdown is irreparable. There are occasions, it must be said, when the patient is in a desperate situation and biotherapies may be too slow to reduce a tumor which is blocking a vital function. In these crisis situations, a conventional procedure would be the choice.

I feel that conventional therapies should be considered only as crisis treatment and used only to the point of reducing the danger of the tumor mass threatening a vital process. Preserving the integrity of the host should be the primary consideration.

BIOLOGICAL REPAIR

I want to reiterate here that the biological healing process requires a coordinated approach that includes nutrition, immune enhancement, stress control, endocrine repair, waste elimination and structural balance. Just as different factors caused the biological breakdown, several corrective treatments may be needed to restore the body's biological integrity.

Needless to say, these biological alternatives are, as of the present, utilized only by a small, growing number of cancer patients and practitioners. Because alternatives are increasingly publicized, and so little understood by the general public, it is imperative to do a serious investigation.

What I have concluded through my experience at FACT, and hope will become the established system, is the implementation of *biologically-sound systems which use the body's natural ability to repair by providing the correct milieu for restoration.* As previously stated, I hope this would be the first choice after surgery before damaging the organism with chemotherapy or radiation in an attempt to achieve tumor reduction.

If a biological repair system is chosen, the goal is to normalize the physical dysfunction—or at least correct it to the level of repair that each person is able to achieve. If the body has reached a point that is irreparable, full recovery may be elusive. Even if recovery is unattainable, benefit is usually derived from improvement in the patient's lifestyle and an extension of quality time is the usual reward. After all, it is beneficial to at least achieve and maintain the highest possible level of health.

More than thirty years ago, to use myself as an illustration, I was a very sick person—taking all sorts of drugs for a host of gastrointestinal problems. I had two benign tumors excised (one in the colon, the other in the breast) and was hospitalized four times for suspected cancer. No one back then would have believed that I would live to be the vigorous, disease-free octogenarian I am today. My condition was chronic and I continued to deteriorate as time went by. In the interim, I changed my lifestyle—diet, attitude and waste elimination habits to improve the general condition of my health. This lifestyle change was responsible for overcoming the chronic struggle I had with health problems. So you see, the body will do all it can to achieve the needed repairs provided you create the correct conditions, give it the kind of guidance it needs and do not obstruct the process of repair.

When one seriously considers the biological approach as a means of encouraging the body's self-healing system, one will need a great deal of understanding, tolerance, a positive attitude toward the therapy, and of course a will to survive and be healthy. The basic element of the treatment is a balanced nutritional program that has all the essential elements required for the production of normal cells. A system of competent waste removal must be put in place as the body replaces abnormal cells with healthy ones and needs to discard the waste. (Aiding the body in the removal of dead cells by specific detoxification techniques, which I will explain in Chapter 6, eases the burden of processing them through the elimination channels.) Severe emotional problems need to be alleviated to reduce stress which plays havoc with the endocrine system, consequently, having a negative effect on metabolism. Avoiding the use of medicines or other substances that have side effects is crucial. Any structural misalignment will require attention or the nerve signals guiding the body's function will be distorted. Any pressure on the nerves may weaken the message from the brain to the organ. One will have to be especially careful to see that the body has all the rest, relaxation, and exercise it needs for self-repair. In these and other ways (which I will discuss at greater length in separate chapters), you have to give your system all the help it requires to repair itself—preferably with the guidance of a biologically-oriented physician.

Some patients are under the impression that their cancer is the result of specific recent damage to the body, such as a fall or an accident. That is most unlikely. Almost always, the precipitating factor occurred years earlier and ended in cancer only because the fall or accident was the straw that broke the camel's back—it allowed what was festering there for a long time to come to the surface. In addition, a visit to the doctor for an injury may reveal the presence of cancer that would have otherwise remained hidden.

In actuality, because of a built-in defense system against disease, a surprising amount of time will elapse before the body breaks down. In Hiroshima, for example, cancer as a consequence of atomic radiation did not appear in some victims until 20 to 30 years from the time the bomb was dropped. It all depends on the individual's constitution and on whether his or her lifestyle is health-giving or disease-causing.

Using a sound alternative system that is suited to the individual can arrest the cancer growth and begin to repair a biological breakdown to the point where the patient is physically comfortable and able to resume a normal, productive life. But if the patient discontinues a program too soon and begins to violate the rules of good health before restoration is complete, usually, the recovery will not be sustained. I have seen this from experience with patients who did extremely well, and then slipped back into their original harmful behavioral patterns. When this occurs, the original biological problems reassert themselves. Most often, it will take about two years for a full repair to take place. I feel it is unwise to ever go back to the disease-causing pattern that was responsible for the illness in the first place. The program can be modified considerably and become one's lifestyle, but it seems foolish to return to an unhealthy way of life.

The success of any biological alternative would benefit greatly from the guidance of a competent practitioner and the conscientiousness of the patient. Practitioners must have training and clinical experience, and understand the different body reactions of each patient, and their unique constitutional endowment. One body starts out with greater strength and potential for healing and controlling disease than another. Some individuals are afflicted with structural or systemic weaknesses that are inherited. With good care and therapeutic assistance, there is no reason why most people (except those that are irreparably damaged) cannot be restored to their optimum level of health. Even when there is inherited weakness to begin with, the body can still function optimally and the individual can be well in mind and body and enjoy living to his or her fullest potential.

I can't possibly spell out in detail what such a therapeutic system would entail for any one person, as everyone has individual strengths and weaknesses. What can be said, however, is that a thorough evaluation can and should be made of each individual's physical condition by their doctor in order to determine his or her particular weaknesses and strengths. These may include such factors as: thyroid function, liver function, kidney function, pancreatic function, blood count (CBC), hormonal balance, waste elimination, and digestive integrity. This evaluation needs to be done carefully for each individual patient, regardless of generalizations that may surface regarding the patient's particular cancer.

DIAGNOSTIC TECHNIQUES

Current diagnostic tools used by conventional medicine and alternative practitioners make these evaluations easily achieved. A Sequential Multiple Analyzer (SMA) evaluation could be a most useful tool. In the alternative arena, iris analysis and Contact Reflex Analysis (CRA), a highly developed form of kinesiology, are tools to provide additional insights. Another effective non-invasive diagnostic technique is an electronic device, known under various names such as Intero and Vega. I was introduced to these originally in Germany where there is much more openness to natural healing than in the United States. The above diagnostic techniques are aimed at providing the practitioner with information about body function to use in designing an individualized biorepair program for the patient.

There are a number of non-invasive diagnostic procedures that are available to a more limited degree. One such procedure, called the Human Chorionic Gonadotrophin (HCG) test, was refined by Emanuel Navarro, M.D., at the University of Santo Tomas in the Philippines. This test provides a quantitative measurement of HCG secretion in the urine, which is linked to cell production. The HCG titre rises relative to cell production, such as with the development of a fetus or at any time there is a need for tissue repair due to a severe burn, surgery or an accident. Dr. Navarro established a measurement of 50 IUs per cc to represent the number for normal cell repair, which is constant. Any rise in the titre, with a lack of the presence of injury or a developing fetus, indicates excess cell production. It is assumed and I feel correctly from my experience with patients, abnormal cells proliferate faster than normal cells. Therefore, a quantitative measurement of the rate of cell production can serve as a guide to monitor a patient, and can also alert the patient of an imminent problem before a tumor is evident.

Since it is important to protect the body against the assaults of foreign materials, one has to consider the effect that certain invasive diagnostic techniques can have on the body, especially x-rays, scans that use radioactive isotopes, or dye that is used to examine the kidney.

I knew a woman who had a barium enema as an x-ray aid, and the barium remained in the colon for many years. During colon surgery performed four years after the barium enema, the surgeon found hardened barium in the colon which was the residue of her earlier enema. The normal body can tolerate much abuse before debilitating effects manifest themselves. But who can estimate how many years are subtracted from one's lifespan? And, of course, where there is already a serious biological impairment, as in cancer, we can be certain that any abuse to the system will hamper the process of repair.

It must be understood that the cancer detection diagnostic procedure now in general use has been dictated by medical officialdom. It is based on the assumption that the biopsy—the excision of a piece of tissue from the living body for diagnosis—is the final determinant of whether or not cancer is present. All other diagnostic techniques, such as mammography or needle biopsy are ordinarily considered preliminary tools. Yet the medical community is aware that the biopsy itself is not always accurate.

We cannot, of course, discard conventional diagnostic techniques either. But they ought to be used with sound judgement and reservation, not more aggressively than is required for the particular problem. As I have pointed out, government health officials have themselves sounded a warning against the overuse of x-rays. There is no point in burdening the human system with more invasive diagnostic work than is absolutely necessary.

There is still another non-invasive procedure called thermography, which is based on measuring the temperature of cancer cells, which are known to be warmer than normal cells. (I am puzzled as to why the medical profession does not use this non-invasive procedure on a broader scale.) It is indeed a safe substitute for mammography, which subjects the tissue to harmful x-rays. There is also the colonoscope, which is used quite extensively, and does not require the barium and x-rays that are needed with other techniques to examine the colon.

I look forward to the day when the medical community will investigate the potential of each of the alternative non-invasive diagnostic procedures, so that they can finally take their place among the diagnostic tools that combine accuracy with safety. Certainly, with time and additional interest, the area of non-invasive diagnoses will be scientifically refined, so that there will be no question about their validity. Hopefully, too, new techniques will be developed with consideration for the biological integrity of the patient.

In the meantime, practitioners and patients alike should consider biologically-sound diagnostic techniques and exercise caution and good judgement when other procedures are necessary. To paraphrase Dr. Bernard Jensen and others who utilize biological concepts of health and disease—the human body ought to be treated like a temple, with the greatest of reverence and respect.

Even the most skilled practitioner cannot be correct one hundred percent of the time, but he or she is better qualified to recognize a flaw and make a needed adjustment than someone without training. Imagine, however, the harm that can be done when amateurs disseminate information, or worse yet, set up a practice to serve cancer patients without being properly prepared.

THE THERAPEUTIC COMPONENTS

When all of the causative factors responsible for the breakdown in body chemistry have been taken into consideration, and every dysfunction put back into working order to the degree possible, the system as a whole can function harmoniously. It should go without saying that every program of biorepair will vary from person to person, in accordance with individual problems and needs.

In the following section, I will present a brief description of the different systems that are available for a health restoration program. Although some of this information has been presented previously I think repetition of the healing processes will impress the importance of it on the reader. It may serve to demonstrate the ways in which the different programs work together, so that if the patient begins to improve his or her nutrition and elimination, and makes the proper corrections in other areas when necessary, the body will respond by improving its overall functioning.

Nutrition

Having said this, I hasten to add that sound nutrition is the primary part of any biological therapy. Our bodies carry on their vital life processes and, indeed, thrive and survive on the basis of the nutritional elements which are supplied to them. Sound nutrition requires that all of the nutrients in adequate amounts and proper balance be present in our food supply for *normal cell production*—the goal we are striving for. For example: Fruits and vegetables are to nourish and cleanse; carbohydrates and fats are major sources of energy; proteins are the building materials for all living cells; enzymes are the catalytic agents which enable the food to be broken down into its microcomponents for cell production. Nature combines vitamins and minerals and enzymes, including trace elements, for competent synergism in order to maintain homeostasis. I have given only the most sketchy and partial description of the various functions which the nutrients perform. They are the most important and most potent elements for producing healthy cells and for restoring health and maintaining it.

Vitamins, Minerals, & Enzymes

The activities of nutrients are interrelated and dependent on Nature's combinations to function at their best. If any of these elements are not present in sufficient quantities, the body will not function at an optimum level. If deprivation continues too long, the body will be unable to keep its cells and organs functioning adequately. A number of deficiency diseases can eventually develop from a chronic biological dysfunction. It is equally true that one can imbalance body chemistry from excess as well as insufficiency. *Overusing* unnecessary vitamin supplements can worsen the very illness you are attempting to cure. There is an assumption pervading the health movement that taking excessive amounts of supplements is alright as the body will eliminate the overload. This is true, except it strains the elimination system, and if the body is handicapped by the surplus it must discard, then it becomes cumulative.

One should not be guided by some fragmented piece of research such as that which has determined a deficiency of zinc, selenium, or any required element is the cause of a rise in cancer and an assumption is then made that using this element is the solution for all cancer patients. Since cancer has multiple causes and other disabilities can be responsible for cancer in some individuals, these one-shot solutions are going to result in failure for most of the patients. I cannot tell you how many times I have seen this piecemeal approach lead to unpredictable symptoms and serious setbacks to the patient's recovery. One individual may have an overload of a vitamin or other nutrient rather than a deficiency. Using the wrong supplement, which was supposed to be good for cancer patients, may exacerbate a problem.

The experienced practitioner can arrange a therapeutic system which takes into consideration all of the problem areas and tries to make corrections to the degree that the patient's body will be able to make that repair. A competent diagnosis, then, combined with proper therapies suited to the patient's physiological needs, are the best assurance that biological balance can be restored.

It is important to take into account, as accurately as possible, the individual's specific nutritional needs, and on this basis arrange a suitable dietary regimen. One should consider, for example, whether the endocrine secretions are available in sufficient quantities to metabolize the food. If not, steps should be taken to correct digestion, absorption and assimilation of nutrients. These steps might include enzyme or glandular supplementation that addresses the particular weakness and deficiency.

It is unwise to make major changes in the diet without guidance unless one has acquired the knowledge needed to understand the physiological changes that can be stimulated and how to handle them constructively. A competently designed, individualized metabolic system is much more potent, much more serious, than most people realize. It is sometimes possible for an individual to institute a change successfully without guidance but it is unusual, therefore risky.

The improvement some people experience on an improved dietary regimen often makes them so enthusiastic that they want their friends, their relatives, the whole world to follow *their* example even though their program may not be applicable to another individual's body chemistry. There may be hundreds of others who make that same change and suddenly find that they suffer from adverse reactions. They may find themselves feeling sicker instead of healthier.

This has happened to cancer patients and others so often that I have devoted Chapter 4 to the dangerous and sometimes frightening effects of incompetent dietary alterations. In that chapter you will find examples from my personal experience with patients that should convince one to exercise caution and preferably consult with a competent guide before instituting a special dietary regimen. I would caution even those people who have degrees in nutrition that their training does not automatically provide the expertise needed to advise the cancer patient during periods of toxicity. Anyone who presumes to give advice on nutrition to cancer patients should have excellent training and experience.

No book can provide a plan or blueprint for personal nutrition—nor should it even attempt to do so. However, I can provide considerable information, gathered from clinical sources and from my experience with thousands of patients and clinicians, on fundamental questions relating to food, nutrition and health. Later on I will discuss in greater detail some of the nutritional therapies that have been used successfully by clinicians and patients. I will begin by providing general information that will be useful to anyone who may need to know more about nutrition.

The purpose of a sound dietary regime is to encourage the body's healing process by correcting nutritional imbalances (deficiencies or excesses). This means that all of the elements—proteins, carbohydrates, fatty acids, vitamins, minerals, trace minerals and, of course, enzymes—must be present in the foods we eat. In addition, the nutrients given to the body should be primarily in their natural state. Vitamins, minerals and enzymes need to be in a complex as Nature designed them, in order to be synergistically sound. In Nature, elements are supplied in a complex; that is, vitamins and minerals are built into the food with their appropriate enzymes. Without enzymes, food cannot be broken down into its microcomponents to be used readily for cell repair and cell production. Man-made supplements cannot duplicate Nature's "formula" adequately; therefore, they should not be routinely considered a healthy substitute for food.

Another important consideration is that the high temperatures used in heating food will inactivate the enzymes, depriving the body of full benefit from the food. That is why a substantial part (not all) of a diet should consist of raw foods. Baked potatoes, beans, squash and other vegetables generally are not consumed in a raw state.

Protein

In any good diet—and particularly in a special nutritional regime for cancer patients—there is a need for adequate amounts of protein. If high protein diets are bad, insufficient protein is equally harmful, as cell growth and repair depends on the presence of this vitally important nutrient. Meat and fish protein sources ought to be of the purest quality, and not be polluted with antibiotics and growth hormones.

Fruits & Vegetables

Sufficient amounts and varieties of fresh vegetables and fruits should be daily constituents of any good dietary regime. Vegetables provide the nourishing elements; the fruits are the cleansers. Both are important, but the vegetables more so. When additional waste removal is necessary, one might add more fruit temporarily to achieve better elimination, then return to the more balanced system. In selecting foods, one must create proper acid/alkaline balance.

Fermented Food

It is essential to include fermented food or lactic acid in the diet. These provide good intestinal flora, and include yogurt, clabbered (sour) milk, some cheese (preferably low-fat, unsalted and raw), quality sauerkraut made without salt (as salt upsets potassium balance), and fermented vegetables made without vinegar.

Oil

We cannot negate oils (fatty acids) as a nutritional requirement. They are a good energy source, act as carriers for vitamins, protect and support the body organs, and structure and form a necessary coating for nerves. Fatty acids can be derived from nuts and avocado or quality cold-pressed oil in moderate quantities. For optimum benefit, oils should never be heated to high temperatures, as occurs when frying foods. Based on the clinical work of Max Gerson, M.D., flaxseed oil is considered the optimal type of oil for the cancer patient.

Whole Grains

Grains in their natural whole state are highly potent in food value. When a seed is planted, it has the whole range of elements necessary to produce a live plant that will produce new seeds to continue propagation. When hot rollers are used to process grains (such as rolled oats) or cooked at a high temperature, they become a dead food. In Chapter 5, you will find a simple way to prepare cereals from whole grains which retains all the natural nutrients without destroying the enzymes through overheating.

Glucose

As you are probably aware, devitalization through overrefining has created a strong anti-sugar sentiment. Many sources espouse the elimination of all sweets, including honey and fruit. But since the cells need glucose—as indeed they need every other nutritional element—such deprivation would cause a deficiency. But where do we get our glucose, and in what quantities? The best way to get glucose is from fresh fruit, and by sweetening some of our foods with raisins or dates, or from raw honey or pure maple syrup.

Refined sugar is a very poor source of glucose. It is addictive and deficient in some of the natural elements because of processing. Avoid foods such as soft drinks, ice cream, pastries, and candies, where sugar is added. (And never use artificial sweeteners in place of sugar.)

Unwholesome Foods

We ought to remove, as much as is humanly possible, the more offensive foods from our diets which are found in supermarkets, and other food outlets. This is easier said than done, since it is virtually impossible to find foods which are entirely free of any additives, pesticides, preservatives, chemicals, carcinogenic hormones, antibiotics, coloring, and other toxins and still maintain a balanced regimen. One should strive to do what one can to keep unwholesome foods to the minimum and compromise only when necessary.

Foods that should be avoided as much as possible are the refined starches such as white rice, spaghetti, cakes, pizzas and most breads. If these refined foods are eaten regularly, the body will have to use up its precious stored nutrients and enzymes in an attempt to make such food synergistic. Preservatives in food kills bacteria, including the healthy colon bacteria (flora) which are needed for waste elimination. There is no reason why people can't become accustomed to eating whole, delicious fresh food instead.

Milk is not an adult food; it was meant by Nature for babies whose bodies provide the enzyme, lactase, which is necessary to metabolize milk. Production of this enzyme begins to wane in the child at about the age of two. On the other hand, fermented milk products, such as clabbered milk, yogurt or cheese, are competently metabolized because the fermentation process is equivalent to predigestion. This fermented material provides healthy intestinal flora that is required by the colon for completion of the end process of eliminating waste from the body.

I pointed out before that an individual with a strong constitution can violate some of the food rules and still live a long, healthy life. This is merely an observation, not an invitation to disregard the principles of sound nutrition. It is important, however, not to make eating an unpleasurable event where people exercise exaggerated care in choosing their food, thereby creating a tense situation that should be avoided. We may have to give up hot dogs, hamburgers, soda pop and white flour products, but there are always better substitutes.

Occasionally, when people have a craving, they may indulge to a limited degree, to avoid feeling deprived. When this occurs, they don't necessarily have to eat foods that can cause damage. Cake, for example, can usually be found in the form of whole grains, instead of refined flour. It isn't the healthiest food, but some people can't seem to eliminate these foods completely from their diets; however, this should never become a consistent part of a dietary regimen.

Naturally, if you are on a strictly regulated nutritional regime, under the care of a professional, and these foods are forbidden, you will just have to do without them. There isn't any food for which you can't find a healthier substitute. When the patient is already in a precarious balance, eating improper foods can be harmful.

A most dramatic example of what can occur was told to me by a practitioner whose seemingly recovered patient celebrated by eating a vast meal of spaghetti and meat sauce, with all the desserts and other trimmings. A few days later he called his doctor to report the reappearance of a tumorous swelling that had disappeared as the result of a good therapeutic regime. Of course, reactions to poor food are ordinarily not this dramatic, but there is no doubt that ill bodies cannot tolerate unwholesome food to the extent that normally healthy people can.

Chemicals in Foods. It is hard to imagine the quantities and varieties of preservatives, chemicals, dyes, fixatives, stabilizers and countless other toxic substances that are sold to and eaten by the average American. Disease statistics underline the tragic effects of this toxic barrage. It is an even greater burden on the cancer patient, who under ideal circumstances should be eating food that is 100% free of toxic chemicals.

If we as consumers demand that these chemicals be left out of food, manufacturers would without doubt provide us with what we want to purchase. It is not too difficult for an aware population to get the Food and Drug Administration (FDA) to protect the food supply from hazardous chemicals. We can get an uncontaminated food supply delivered to us instead of struggling so hard to find unpoisoned foods. In a discussion I had with an official of the Food and Drug Administration, as I wanted to be included in a nutritional conference, I suggested that the subject of additives be placed on the agenda. The official responded by saying that there was only a minute amount of these chemicals allowed in foods. She claimed that it would take a hundred years before a buildup could occur that would be harmful. I pointed out that in an already sick body plagued by faulty waste elimination, poisons in food become cumulative and cannot be removed efficiently. I also pointed out that this answer does not take into account the fact that these same chemicals can be used in more than one food, and that one individual can be consuming the same additive from ten or more different products. Under these circumstances, the hundred years that it takes for the accumulation to become dangerous to the human system is then reduced to ten or even fewer years.

One must also consider the effect on the body from receiving a variety of chemicals from many different food sources. Although drugs have been tested extensively, doctors have to be extremely careful about combining medications as the interaction can be deadly; the combination of chemicals found in food products can be equally dangerous.

Stress Reduction

Tension, extreme mental agitation and other negative patterns of behavior are a troublesome area which must be attended to if one wants to stay well or if one is involved in a recovery program. Chronic tension, as we have noted, activates a stress mechanism which can overwork the endocrine glands and immune system, and lead to exhaustion and greater susceptibility to organ impairment and disease.

One of the most serious consequences of this overactivated stress mechanism is that it cuts down on the efficiency of food metabolism and waste elimination. Even with a healthy diet, if the digestive juices are not secreted properly because stress has skewed the process, the body will have difficulty breaking down the nutrients into the microcomponents necessary for normal cell production. If the conditions under which one lives are not conducive to controlling the stress factors, then one has to use special techniques to overcome the negative impact of stress on the body. If this is not done, the patient is going to fail with his or her biological repair program. Biofeedback and meditation, as well as other stress reduction techniques, are outstanding methods for minimizing the impact on the body. Counseling or any other technique for calming your mind and getting your body into a state of relaxation also would be beneficial. Often one cannot change basic attitudes, but biofeedback or meditation can give the body the respite it needs from physiological damage caused by continuing stress.

Using drugs to alleviate stress can introduce complications that may interfere with the body's ability to control cancer or other health problems. The causes of stress should not be controlled by drugs; biofeedback or meditation may safely relieve its overstimulating impact on the body.

Any serious and long-term ailment, whether it is cancer or other degenerative diseases, places tremendous psychological and physical pressure on the patient and, of course, the family. It is therefore essential that we create an atmosphere for ourselves where tension, anxiety and depression do not interfere with the healing process. Near the conclusion of this book you will find a number of actual case histories of individuals who recovered from cancer. When you read their moving stories, I think you will be impressed by the common qualities they all share—tremendous courage, positive attitude and determination to survive and stay well despite all of the setbacks they encountered.

Physical Fitness

It is hard to imagine a valid system of therapy that neglects the importance of physical fitness and does not include some form of gentle, limbering exercise or other conditioning activity. Naturally, the amount of activity will depend on the condition of each patient. But most people, whatever their age, can raise the level of their fitness in any number of ways: from taking long walks to practicing deep breathing techniques, from improving one's posture to engaging in physical exercise, from enjoying hobbies like gardening or golf to using a slant board for sit-ups and stretching.

This should be a part of our life pattern—not merely a temporary aspect of a health restoration program. It will pay back more immediate and long-term benefits than I can list here. It can tone the muscles and increase musculoskeletal strength; enhance stamina; improve oxygen intake; improve circulation, thereby bringing more nutrients to the cells and stimulating better waste removal; and decrease stress and its symptoms. And, getting more in touch with yourself and your environment can help develop a more life-affirming attitude.

Sleep and Relaxation

One health factor, given only minor attention that should be considered an essential component of any biological repair regime, is adequate sleep. People have a tendency to violate this particular biological need of their bodies. They will interrupt their sleep even though it is what the body demands and needs at the time, just as a hungry body demands that it be fed. If the body is fatigued and wants sleep or rest, it should be listened to, because it is fulfilling one of Nature's vital needs. Despite this, people have a way of avoiding or postponing sleep to read, watch television or even finish work. As a result, they may rely on an alarm clock to awaken them before they are refreshed in order to carry on the day's activities. This interruption is unhealthy. Each arousal from deep sleep—particularly if it is sudden—interferes with the healing process that takes place during sleep. Not to give your body the sleep it wants is another abuse of natural law that can drain the vital life energies essential for overcoming disease. For an in-depth exploration of the harm of sleep deprivation and how to alleviate it, I recommend the book, *The Promise of Sleep* by William Dement, M.D.

In addition to regular sleep, the human organism needs periodic times set aside for rest, relaxation and leisure to renew its energies for physical and mental well-being. Time used for recreation, meditation, holidays away from home, communing with nature, sunbathing, reading or listening to music—or even doing nothing at all—are as important a part of getting well as are physical activities. For cancer patients, who tend to be under greater stress than most people, learning to let go and relax is a vital part of therapy.

Addictive Habits

One would not ordinarily think that it would be necessary to warn patients about the dangers of harmful addictions such as coffee, tea, alcohol and other habit-forming drugs. Yet I know individuals who faithfully follow rigorous nutritional and elimination therapies, but at the same time continue destructive old habits which in themselves may have been causative factors in their illness.

I am not speaking of an occasional smoke, or the uncontrollable urge to take a cup of coffee, tea, chocolate drinks or milk. I mean people who (secretly, for the most part) continue to make coffee part of their dietary pattern, even though they may know that caffeine in sufficient quantities (like smoking) can accumulate in the body as dangerous toxins. Sleeplessness, bad nerves, overacidity, heartburn—these are only a few of the damages that can result from habitual caffeine consumption. A number of research studies have confirmed this high correlation between caffeine and disease. When the coffee urge occurs, wouldn't it be a better idea to drink herbal teas, fruit juices or other biologically-sound substitutes that add to your nutritional health rather than drain your body?

Spinal Manipulation

If there are stresses along the spinal column, spinal manipulation may be needed to clear the nerve pathways. Otherwise, there will be a disruption of signals sent to the organs that must be working for your body to function harmoniously. As I previously indicated, among the problems that can result from this interference with the autonomic system are poor digestion and poor waste elimination. These in turn will undo some of the benefits of the best therapuetic program.

Temporomandibular Joint (TMJ)

Without an experienced practitioner to guide them, most people don't take the potential danger of temporomandibular joint (TMJ) blockage into account. It is wise to incorporate structural integrity into a therapeutic program with the help of an osteopath or chiropractor. Structural integrity should include the temporomandibular joint (TMJ). One has to see that there is no misalignment of the jaw joint (the two joints in front of the ears where the lower jaw hinges). If one or both of these joints is out of position, circulation and nerve signals tend to be blocked.

Most dentists and doctors rarely relate multiple symptoms of a chronic nature with stress brought about by TMJ problems. However, if there is a problem, efficient realignment of the jaw joint can be made by cranial adjustments. A more permanent correction can be made by a dentist trained in TMJ adjustments. When the displacement of the joint is corrected, it creates an opportunity for circulation to normalize in the cranial area. I have known correction of the TMJ to relieve hearing loss, tinnitus and macular degeneration. Alleviating the blockage of the nerves and arteries allows nourishment to circulate to the deprived areas, arresting the degenerative process.

Detoxification

I hope it is evident to the reader by now that no therapeutic system—which includes the finest nutritional substances—is going to be effective unless the waste (elimination) system is functioning normally and wastes are constantly being cleared from the body.

Waste products deposited in a healthy colon with good musculature will be carried to the anal area and eliminated from the bowels sometimes two or three times a day. When, however, the colon has poor muscle tone, the waste products remain there—sometimes for long periods of time. This could lead to all kinds of functional problems and metabolic breakdowns.

The human system is strong and resilient; it tolerates many abuses and still goes on to maintain life, although that may not be at its most energetic level. In order to truly restore health, particularly from a degenerative disease such as cancer, the body's repair processes must be encouraged in every possible way.

A carefully designed, individualized metabolic regime is the most effective means of bringing about health restoration. But to optimize the effects of nutritional improvement, detoxification must be an integral part of the repair program. Better nutrition without including waste removal techniques can bring about unpredictable and very unpleasant health problems.

Eliminating the system's toxic wastes is the essence of any detoxification therapy. The colon should be kept clean on a daily basis. Internal cleanliness is more important than external cleanliness. Allowing the waste from meal after meal to remain in the colon for two, three or more days is like keeping garbage in the garbage pail too long. It putrefies. The toxins in these wastes will be absorbed into the bloodstream through the portal vein. The bloodstream will be cleaned out as much as possible by the liver and the waste sent back once again to the colon. If it is not eliminated with the help of the colon musculature or cleansing, it will be recirculated. You can visualize what can happen—and what actually does happen—to the system if this process repeats itself. It exhausts the elimination system and contributes to an imbalance in the whole body chemistry.

I say this not only on the basis of study and feedback from many patients, but through my own discussions with some of the best practitioners in the United States, Canada and Europe, who include detoxification as a major part of their biological repair programs. No matter how careful we are, however, I don't think any of us is going to have perfect colon elimination all the time—there are simply too many poisons in the foods, air and water. But we can do a great deal in spite of this to see that our waste products are properly eliminated.

Among the most effective detoxification procedures are enemas and colonics. There are, in addition, a number of other waste elimination techniques which I shall describe in Chapter 6. In this area, as indeed elsewhere, I cannot advise individuals what procedures are best for their particular needs. That is up to the patient, possibly with the doctor's cooperation. What I can do, however, is inform you that detoxification as part of an overall repair program has helped many patients restore their health.

Organ Repair

The question as to what can be done to repair a damaged or weak organ is one that arises very often and is frequently misunderstood. Orthodox medicine, with its emphasis on highly specialized areas, tends to view and treat each organ, whether it is a liver or the kidneys, as a separate entity, rather than as one link in a chain of organs whose functions are interconnected and affect one another constantly. The patient is therefore given a diagnostic work-up which presumably tells the physician that the liver is healthy or unhealthy; the lungs are fine or diseased; the thyroid is sound or unsound, and so forth. The diagnoses do not indicate, however, if there are minor weaknesses which can gradually deprive the body of good health.

If one is going to utilize the system of biorepair, the point is not to isolate the problem of one particular organ and seek to repair just that organ. This is precisely the approach which conventional medicine takes. The direction, rather, should be to try to use as many biological repair techniques as are indicated in order to get all of the organs to function synergistically—at least to the degree that they can. Hopefully, this level of activity will be adequate to overcome a diseased state and restore good health.

When I refer to a breakdown in body chemistry, almost any organ or combination of organs can be involved. If one organ is impaired, other organs tend to compensate for the weakness as best they can. Sometimes, however, organs become overexhausted, causing the body to manifest a state of ill health.

These are not just assumptions or theoretical concepts. They are part of an overall concept behind the research and clinical work done by Dr. John H. Tilden, Dr. Harvey Kellogg, Dr. William Howard Hay, Dr. Max Gerson, Dr. Bernard Jensen, Dr. Norman W. Walker, Dr. Max Warmbrand, Dr. Are Waerland and many other nutritional pioneers here and in Europe. This approach is aimed at helping the whole body repair itself rather than attempting a piecemeal solution—such as attempting to deal with the tumor or any other symptom of chronic disease. Only in this systemic way, the practitioners felt, could they get the entire body to function smoothly and in harmonious interrelationship.

None of these practitioners makes the claim that the biological repair system is a direct treatment for cancer. At its most effective, it helps the body do its own repair work. This is by no means a new idea; it goes back to the time of Hippocrates, who wrote: "Let food be thy medicine." It is an idea being accepted, or at least listened to attentively, by an increasing number of physicians and scientists.

I have spoken about the ways in which nutrition can provide the body with the nutrients needed to aid the repair process. Our bodies are made from food and sustained by food. Any improvement in the body is bound to be reflected as an overall improvement in the body's organs, tissues and cells. In this vital sense, better nutrition and waste elimination can be considered primary tools for organ repair.

When one organ is not working normally, the body as a whole can be affected. Science and medicine have been investigating the intricacies of organs, tissue and cells—down to the nucleic material in the cells on a molecular and even submolecular level—instead of concentrating on the overall function of the organism. Some remarkable scientific research has been done on this fundamental level—some of which I sincerely believe confirms the biological concepts that we support. Too often medicine as it is now practiced loses sight of the body as a whole and the integrated way in which all of the cells, tissues and organs relate to and affect each other's functions. I hope and expect that the future direction of medicine will be an integrated system that encompasses the whole body.

I have discussed a series of factors that must be taken into account in any program for maintaining health or restoring health to the degree that is possible in each individual. It is only natural that people place the most emphasis in the area where they experience the greatest difficulty. One places it on the stress factor; another on nutrition, or of course on the organ where there is a demonstrated pathology. What I am trying to do here is to avoid putting undue emphasis on any one area, so that the patient can take an overall view that stress, nutrition, waste removal, structural balance, and a sound attitude toward life must all get attention—and that no one problem need be emphasized to the neglect of another. When all of these factors are evaluated and normalized, it is *possible to achieve a state of biological integrity which can be defined as good health.*

4. The Symptoms Associated with Biological Repair

*Good instincts usually tell you what to do
long before your head has figured it out.*
—MICHAEL BURKE

Many people have the mistaken belief that a biorepair is a simple procedure that can be undertaken on one's own without any guidance. This is an assumption which unfortunately is fostered by health books and magazines, by well-meaning but inexperienced people, and even by patients who pass along a particular form of biological therapy that worked for them. On occasion this may work, but when it does not, the consequences can be disastrous.

I can remember when I was first introduced to better nutrition and my great enthusiasm for its benefit. At that time, I had little knowledge of the complications that could ensue in the wake of physiological changes. Today, after three decades of active work at FACT, conferences with top-grade practitioners, and feedback from cancer and other patients, I am fully aware of the incredible complexity of the biorepair process and the unforeseeable reactions that can be provoked by changes in body chemistry associated with healing.

The best I can do is present what I have investigated carefully and learned from personal contact with thousands of patients. The symptoms they experienced from what I have termed "the housecleaning process" ranged anywhere from a slight cold, headaches, nausea, to rashes, fever, diarrhea and bleeding. These are signs that the body was trying to eliminate the stored accumulation of foreign material that could have been responsible for their present condition of ill health. It is a time when a person needs experienced guidance, or the healing process may overwhelm the body's ability to eliminate the waste effectively and thus produce the stressful symptoms of autointoxication. (Autointoxication occurs when the body's fluids become overloaded with toxins.) Only with knowledge and experience in the biorepair processes can these unpredictable and unexpected symptoms be resolved comfortably. Dr. Max Gerson referred to these healing phases as "flare ups."

One of the most difficult things for me to explain to people is why they get these distressing symptoms as the result of a repair that is supposed to help them get well. And yet it is a rare situation for someone to undertake a biorepair program, including superior nutrition and immune enhancement, without going through unusual reactions as the body adjusts to the new internal milieu and lifestyle. This is the physiology of healing. It is the wisdom of the body.

In this chapter I will report some of the complications that can manifest and why they are nearly always inevitable, but useful. Many individuals have been led to believe that these symptoms occur only when you improve your diet; it is not only better nutrition but, anything that improves the healing capability of the body, as is the result of any procedure that enhances vitality such as lymphatic massage. Any debris stored in the lymphatics would be treated by the body as foreign material. Improving the body's healing capability would start the elimination cycle. Any system that enhances the body's healing energy will stimulate the movement of wastes out of storage—from the lymphatics, tissue, colon, and intestinal wall. These methods include stress control, cell therapy, immune activators, osteopathic or chiropractic manipulation.

It is essential for an individual to be aware of what can happen when using a specific biorepair therapy. Otherwise, being ignorant of what to expect, the patient can be disconcerted and on occasion even panicked when an unusual symptom shows up. Discharges might manifest as nose bleeds, diarrhea, excessive sweating, runny nose, phlegm, or coughing. If the individual cannot tolerate these symptoms, knowing in advance what they might be, it is preferable not to initiate a repair program at all. There is good reason why we at FACT want to encourage the medical community to become involved in biorepair. Patients need access to professional guidance and supervision, and when unfamiliar changes occur, reassurance that the cancer is not becoming more aggressive and running rampant. With the guidance of an experienced practitioner, the task of travelling through the ups and downs of healing can be physically and emotionally comfortable.

SYMPTOMS OF CHANGE

Why then does the human body respond to a biological therapy, which is meant to improve its healing ability, by producing a broad spectrum of distressing symptoms? The answer is to be found in the amazing intelligence with which Nature has endowed every cell, tissue and organ system, and in the body's inherent desire and capacity to restore homeostasis when it is given the opportunity to do so.

This natural healing instinct is evident whenever you provoke a biological change—as through better nutrition. The blood carries the quality nutrients to the cell and washes away the stored waste material which is now being discarded because previously the body lacked the vitality to eliminate sufficiently. The healthier cells begin to throw out all kinds of wastes which may have been stored for a long time.

The body originally places the wastes in storage as part of its innate attempt to maintain normal function. They are kept there so that, hopefully, under normal circumstances they can be released through the normal channels of elimination (colon and kidneys) instead of collecting in the tissues and glands.

When the body finds an opportunity to rid itself of these offensive toxins, it may trigger distressful symptoms, among them bad breath, gas, fever, nausea, and frequent bowel movements. The body will also try to rid itself of excess toxins through other body apertures.

Another, more dramatic, analogy may explain why the body feels ill when it is undergoing a healing change. Most of us are familiar with the condition of a drug addict when he goes "cold turkey." As long as he continues to take drugs, he feels calm and quiet. This is because the continuous use of drugs suppresses the healing action, thus maintaining the debris (toxins) in storage. But when the drugs are removed and no longer suppress elimination, the stored drugs flood the bloodstream and the body undergoes withdrawal symptoms which are very uncomfortable. The nose runs, eyes tear, there will be shaking, internal pains and other external manifestations of difficulties. This is caused by the release of toxins into the bloodstream to be processed for elimination through normal channels. Admittedly, this is an extreme situation. However, when you introduce any technique to stimulate the repair process, the body will utilize its own unpredictable devices to eliminate whatever has overloaded the system and obstructed normal functioning.

Since nutrition is *the most potent tool* of biorepair, let me elaborate on what happens in your body when you provide it with better nutrition. Given food of a higher quality, the body gratefully begins to absorb the superior nutrients, which are needed for the life processes, and discards the waste materials from its cells. These toxic wastes may include stored proteins, excess sugar, salt or caffeine, worn-out cells that need to be replaced, abnormal cells, drug deposits and chemical pollutants from the air, food and water.

As the bloodstream brings the better materials to the cells, where they are eagerly absorbed, the stored wastes are discarded. Since the blood washes the cells, the bloodstream may become quite polluted with the toxins it is now carrying away. It is in this interim period, before the liver clears the toxins from the bloodstream, that the body will produce the symptoms I have described. I cannot spell out all of the forms these reactions can take. Acne, shingles, boils, colds, and fever are all symptoms that the body is in a "housecleaning" mode. The fever is the wisdom of the body causing it to rest so that the energy usually expended for a normal day's activity can be used for healing.

The Release of Wastes

Since the normal process of the body is for the liver to cleanse foreign substances from the bloodstream, these toxic wastes are dumped through the bile duct into the intestinal system, where they will end up in the bowel for elimination. Some of the toxins will also be filtered for elimination by the kidneys. But if the waste is flowing faster than the body can completely eliminate it through the colon and kidneys, it will find other avenues for release. The lungs will bring up some of this waste in the form of mucous. If the toxins reach the skin—another large and wonderful organ of elimination— they can be sweated out through the pores or cause a skin rash, or boil.

Although it happens rarely, bleeding through the nose is another reaction by the body to relieve itself of toxicity. Still another occurrence, although rarer, is blood in the stool or urine. This usually comes about as drainage from the lymphatic system, which has the burden of temporarily collecting and holding some of the toxicity to relieve the bloodstream. As soon as conditions allow, the lymphatics return the waste back to the bloodstream where they are processed by the liver for complete elimination. The body is an intelligent organism. Heed its wisdom!

Here is an interesting example: A woman melanoma patient called me very late one evening to tell me that a lump on the back of her knee the size of an orange was bleeding profusely. She was letting it bleed onto a towel which by now was soaked with the blood-like material. I suggested that, to be safe, she make arrangements with her doctor so that if she was actually hemorrhaging, she could enter a hospital for a possible transfusion. We were on the telephone until three o'clock in the morning, because she was afraid if she fell asleep she might bleed to death during the night.

At some point in our long conversation, I asked her if she felt any weakness from the bleeding, and she answered that there was no lessening of energy of any kind. I suggested to her that there was no evidence that this was a hemorrhage, since by this time she would be feeling faint. One can sever an artery and bleed to death before getting to the hospital if it isn't handled properly, but in this instance there was no loss of vitality at all. I suggested to her that it was probably lymphatic fluid draining from the tumor. Somewhat calmer, she decided to go to sleep. The next morning she called to tell me that she felt no worse, and that she had wrapped a Pamper around the discharging area to collect the seepage. What she began to do after that was to use fresh Pampers, each morning and evening. Each time the Pamper was removed it was soaked with the red substance, which to a lay person's eye would appear to be blood. At no time during this period—which continued for thirty days—was there any lessening of energy, so the substance leaking onto the Pamper actually was not blood. When the seepage finally stopped after 30 days, a lump she had in the groin and the one behind the knee flattened, and the woman felt a resurgence of normal energy.

A different kind of lymphatic reaction occurred to another woman who was afflicted with widespread adenocarcinoma. One night, she frantically called her doctor, who had been referred to her by FACT, to inform him that dark, plug-like masses and other very thick material were coming out of her nose and uncontrollable elimination was taking place from the bowel. She had been on a stringent nutritional and waste-elimination program and had been improving very gradually.

The doctor rushed over to her home in time to take a two-inch-long dark-colored plug from her nostril which turned out to be a viscous mucosal material. After a while, the elimination of the same kind of thick substance from her bowels subsided as well. A few days later, a number of tumorous swellings on her skull, neck and shoulders had almost entirely gone down. Evidently, the cleansing of the waste materials had allowed the body to hasten the repair process to the point where it could begin to deal with the tumors.

Another symptom that can understandably cause the patient to panic occurs when the lungs fill up with wastes which are coughed up through the throat. Without the guidance of an experienced person, there may be an immediate assumption that the symptom is a metastatic spreading of the cancer cells—to the lungs. I know of other situations where patients with bone cancer who were on a repair program began to suffer severe aches and pains in their bones and jumped to the conclusion that it was the result of a metastasis to the bones. This may not, in fact, be the case at all. It may be a symptomatic manifestation of the bone reabsorbing better nutritional minerals.

The illustrations I have given above are all aspects of a repair process that needs exposure and understanding. They do not ordinarily occur to the serious extent that I have described above, but the individual who chooses to undertake a biological therapy has to be prepared if unpredictable and unfamiliar things happen. The compensation for these symptoms is the knowledge that they are by-products of the body throwing off toxic accumulation, thereby increasing its capacity to effect a repair of the patient's biological breakdown.

A Rise in Temperature

Sometimes the body reacts to biological changes by means of a rise in temperature. I recall an incident where a patient with lymphosarcoma began to run a temperature of 105°F. It had been stimulated by a metabolic program. He was under the care of his son, a first-year medical school student who had access to medical information any time he needed it. Ordinarily, the next step would be to call a doctor who would no doubt use an antibiotic. The antibiotic would not only have added more foreign material to the body, but would have repressed the symptoms by bringing down the fever. When the fever did not go down by itself, I introduced the son to Dr. Robert A. Berman, who had done extensive research into systemic thermotherapy, sometimes referred to as fever therapy or wholebody hyperthermia. Dr. Berman had designed the water-filled blankets that were heated to artificially raise body temperature.

No one knows for certain why fever, a natural phenomenon, assists in the healing process. At least one government agency—the National Institute of Allergy and Infectious Diseases (NIAID)—had previously done research and concluded that fever is a natural healing process rather than a disease process. Hyperthermia has been used experimentally in a number of hospitals as a means of destroying cancer cells. In some European clinics, fever has been utilized extensively for many years by natural healers and physicians. I presented this information to the lymphoma patient's son, and explained why fever was not something he should fear and rush to suppress. As a matter of fact, in systemic hyperthermia, body temperature is raised as high as 107.5°F. The advantage of systemic hyperthermia is that it destroys malignant cells without harming normal cells. I cannot understand why systemic thermotherapy has not been adopted as a routine practice in the treatment of cancer.

After consulting together, the son, with Dr. Berman's guidance, decided to let the fever run its course, watching carefully to see that there was no injury to the patient. The fever stayed at about 105°F for approximately 10 days, and at the end of this period the glandular swellings disappeared. "It was a miracle," said his son, who is now a practicing physician. This was a patient in the fourth stage of lymphoma, which meant there was limited time he was expected to live using conventional therapy. Knowing what the prognosis was for his father, the son was willing to try the biological process first. After the fever subsided, the patient was put on a very light juice diet, and no other medication at all. Nature and *skilled guidance* did the rest.

Fever plays an important role in the healing process. Interferon* is a biological substance that is used in conventional immunotherapy. Any immune enhancer usually causes a rise in temperature and flu-like symptoms that are obvious symptoms of "housecleaning." Fever is Nature taking control of healing by putting the body at "bed rest" so that its energy can be diverted to healing and detoxification.

---

*Interferon is a natural healing substance that the healthy body produces by itself if the immune system is functioning normally. It seems to be present in insufficient quantities in the blood of cancer patients. When it is given to the patient, his or her revitalized immune system will use it to encourage the body to rid itself of any material which it considers foreign. These are wastes—whether they be cast-off cells or a toxic chemical bioaccumulation.

Unfortunately, instead of trying to nurture the rise in temperature and allowing the fever to subside on its own when it has finished its elimination effort, physicians too often resort to routine protocol and use antibiotics to curb the very healing process that the immunotherapy has stimulated. It would be far better, in most circumstances, to let the fever run its course under supervision, or else, when necessary to use cold liquids or other techniques for cooling the body if the temperature rises too high. This is why we look forward to the time when more members of the medical profession will become actively involved in dealing with the biological repair methods I have been discussing. Their experienced guidance would be invaluable.

As you can see, in all of the above situations, the decisions were made by the individuals themselves; a doctor was on call, and a hospital was available for emergencies. Under these circumstances the patient is not at risk. Each individual has to decide for himself or herself just what he or she wants to do. I can only inform patients and practitioners, based on my vast experience, the knowledge that I have acquired during my years in an organization committed to biorepair and my extensive contact with patients and outstanding practitioners worldwide.

A Healing Concept for All Patients

The process which produces some of the symptoms I have described occurs not only in cancer patients, but in individuals who utilize a biorepair system for any ailment. Even in a person who is apparently in good health but wants to effect improvements, choosing a biological repair system will stir up changes, and these have to be recognized. A one-day juice fast, for instance, can on occasion provoke such typical healing symptoms as bad breath, a headache, a slight fever, a rash, unusual sweating, or diarrhea.

Depending on one's condition, the kind and amount of wastes being discarded and the particular biological therapy, symptoms will vary from person to person. Some people experience very mild reactions, such as a small drop in energy, a chill or temporary sluggishness of the bowel movement. Or the process can do the opposite and cause diarrhea, in addition to irritability, a letdown feeling, or restlessness. The same or other symptoms may appear in a more severe form when there is extreme weakness of the eliminatory organs.

One cannot tell in advance how an individual is going to react to an immune stimulator. Even a very small change in one's dietary pattern can evoke a strong reaction in some people. This is the reason why we have to caution people from altering their nutritional habits without the help of competent guidance, or at least acquire their own in-depth knowledge. Because of my years of experience, I am always disturbed by attempts at healing by people not properly trained. (The old adage, "A little knowledge is a dangerous thing" is absolutely applicable in this instance.)

As a matter of fact, I spoke recently to a doctor who has a great deal of experience in biological repairs, and he told me of a situation that illustrates graphically what can happen when people make basic dietary changes without professional advice or understanding. A patient informed him that she had recently been diagnosed as having leukemia, and was experiencing a number of extremely distressing symptoms. She asked about an alternative therapy and was told that it included a nutritional regime. To his astonishment, she revealed that she had been on a nutritional system which a friend had suggested—it consisted almost entirely of raw vegetable juices. The doctor's feeling was, and I concurred, that the juice diet had stirred up so many toxins in her system that they had invaded the bloodstream and caused the distressing reaction. This unfortunate experience turned her against any further consideration of a nutritional program.

It is not nutrition alone that can stimulate disturbing healing symptoms, but it also can happen when correcting structural misalignments. Sometimes, osteopathic or chiropractic manipulation, or even an ordinary massage, can encourage a cleansing reaction. These symptoms are not anything to be alarmed about. On the contrary, they are happening because the therapy has helped the body release some of its stored toxins, and the system is taking this opportunity to finally eliminate them. Until they can be eliminated through the bowel, kidneys, skin or lungs, the toxic materials can temporarily provoke physical discomfort.

Recently, I referred an acquaintance of mine to a doctor who is known to be one of the nation's experts in stress control through biofeedback. My friend had complained of severe muscular tension, a palpitating heart, bad nerves and sleeplessness, to the point where normal living was all but impossible. After several weeks of concentrated biofeedback techniques, his muscles began to relax, his pulse went down to normal, and he slept through the night for the first time in years. Yet, he called back only a few days later to tell me that he was once again feeling tense, his nerves were jumpy, he had lost his appetite, and he had diarrhea. Should he stop the biofeedback therapy, he asked, and try some other form of treatment?

I explained to him that the biofeedback had encouraged his body to release some excess toxicity that was responsible for the wear and tear on his body and emotional state. As a result of the biofeedback, his muscles had relaxed, his digestive juices were now functioning more normally, and nutrients were assimilated to the point where they were more available to the cells. This in turn enabled the body to give up more of its stored wastes, which were being discarded faster than his eliminatory system could handle. The symptoms were by-products of this process, a sign that his body was now able to cleanse itself of wastes that had been present in the tissues for a long time. In short, the very success of the repair process had paradoxically caused some of his original symptoms to return. My friend went back to his stress management doctor, in the realization that the reoccurrence of symptoms was the small price he would have to pay for gradually correcting a chronic stress condition which had been seriously undermining his health.

Once the body has "cleaned house" it can begin to function more normally. When, for example, the blocked signals to organs are cleared up, the result is an improvement in a number of organ functions, including circulation. The digestive system will be able to metabolize food more efficiently, and waste will be eliminated instead of being stored.

Any biological improvement—change in lifestyle, realigning the temporomandibular joint, structural manipulation, stress management to calm the nerves, even simple exercises to improve muscle tone—can cause physiological reactions.

I hope I have emphasized sufficiently that it is best to undertake a repair program with competent guidance, or at least adequate knowledge of the process. Every system brings into play a different set of body reactions, from a minor rash to a high fever. The novice is not going to be able to determine whether the symptoms that appear are healing reactions or the progression of disease. The best thing one can do, in these situations, is to treat the symptoms as if they were by-products of toxicity that the healing technique had brought on. If the reaction subsides in a few days, the individual will know this was the actual case and not a worsening of a disease condition.

Only a competent professional will be able to evaluate the patient's vital signs, allay his or her fears if complications arise, and make an informed decision as to what needs attention. These are compelling reasons, indeed, to encourage the medical community to become more actively involved in the biorepair system and be available to serve patients who need their help.

During the time that a patient is involved in a biological therapy regimen, it is important to get sufficient rest and sleep, carry out the prescribed detoxification procedures efficiently, and remain in a serene state. It is also important to realize that healing is never a straightforward and uninterrupted process, and that symptoms can reappear any time the patient undergoes a biological change. Disconcerting as these reactions can be, keep in mind they are temporary and should not be avoided. They are Nature's way of flushing out toxins to achieve a state of better health.

5. Balanced Nutrition for Better Health

*An ordinary pig knows more about diet than
the most learned college professor.*
—J. HARVEY KELLOGG, M.D.

When FACT was established in 1971, the prevailing opinion was that there was no connection between diet and cancer and to even suggest so was a form of quackery! In the ensuing decades, however, more and more scientific evidence has indicated there is a link. It is no longer considered unusual when government and private agencies, as well as scientific institutions, publicly confirm the role nutrition plays in cancer and other degenerative diseases. On the contrary, barely a week goes by these days when the media does not trumpet the newly discovered miraculous anti-cancer qualities of some common everyday food which may contradict the previous week's reporting. The effect on the public has been, and is, rampant confusion.

As only one of many examples, an official publication of the American Cancer Society noted that colon and breast cancer show clear evidence of being related to nutrition—too much fat—and accounts for more than half of all cancer. A Joint Senate Investigating Committee stated that the hundreds of chemicals and adulterants in the food—most of which were never fully tested—were one of the chief causes of cancer. And the Canadian Cancer Society recommended the need for a well-balanced diet on the basis of increasing evidence that the state of our nutrition may play a role in causing cancer.

I find it heartening that the principal tenet of the biorepair concept has won some measure of official recognition. We have long been aware, however, that better nutrition goes beyond merely being a preventive measure. From the earliest part of the twentieth century, there have been many—doctors and other health practitioners, particularly in Europe—who treated degenerative diseases, including cancer, nutritionally with excellent results. On the basis of my own experience, I have seen that a balanced nutritional program (one that provides all the elements necessary to build healthy cells, enhances immunity and corrects any physiological impairment) has produced the best long-term results in restoring the health of cancer patients. Isn't it logical? The body is made of cells; cells are made of nutrients. I look forward to the time, hopefully not too far off, when it will be recognized within the medical profession as a whole that nutrients, when competently metabolized, are an effective therapeutic tool in producing healthy cells, and are necessary in the treatment of cancer.

Better nutrition consists of providing the body with high quality foods in proper balance. I define "proper balance" as a condition in which all of the essential nutrients—proteins, carbohydrates, minerals, oils (fatty acids), glucose, sodium, vitamins and enzymes—are present in sufficient quantity and quality to produce healthy cells. This includes everything from digesting and metabolizing the foods, to building and repairing the tissues, to eliminating waste from the body. On the other hand, unbalanced nutrition brought on by dietary deficiencies or excesses, unwholesome foods or organ impairment may contribute to a debilitating biological breakdown.

Because of the great hunger and need for nutritional information, and the importance of clearing up some dangerous misconceptions, this chapter will be devoted to a discussion of the basic principles underlying the nutritional approach. I want to emphasize once again, however, that my purpose is entirely educational, and that it would be injudicious for cancer patients to make dietary changes without the guidance of an experienced person. Only the trained person who has worked with many cancer patients, and is familiar with a wide variety of cancer types, is competent to design a nutritional regime that is suited to the individual's physical condition and specific health needs.

FOODS TO AVOID

The first step on the path to better nutrition is the elimination of poor quality and chemically-altered food. Fifty years ago, the foods we purchased and ate were far more simple, natural and less processed than they are today. Because of this current excessive processing, a great many of our food products are devitalized and, consequently, largely deficient in vitamins, minerals, especially enzymes, and other nutrients. Processing of white sugar, white flour, and white rice have removed much of the natural elements that are necessary for competent metabolism. Some grains have been milled and refined to the point where they have lost too much of their nutritional value and are therefore not synergistically sound. If, for instance, the outer hull or germ is removed from wheat, you have a fragmented material, not as Nature originally supplied it; the essential nutrients are no longer working together for efficient metabolism.

Other foods that cannot be considered part of an improved dietary program are refined starches such as: pasta, pastries and most breads. We should also try to avoid the kinds of overprocessed and preserved products which are sometimes termed "junk food." These include candies, cookies, commercial ice creams, soda pop, potato chips, etc. And, of course, packaged and convenience products that are stacked on the supermarket shelves as "fast foods" are rarely nutritious. As far as habituating substances such as coffee and tea are concerned, they are overstimulating to the nervous system. There are perfectly good substitutes which are far healthier, such as herbal teas. We should also drink distilled water, which does not contain chemicals (chlorine or fluoride) or other pollutants. I don't think we need to dwell too much on the destructive qualities of alcohol.

It should be emphasized, too, that many people have been consuming quantities of animal protein above and beyond what the body can comfortably metabolize. We need to be reminded, for example, that excess protein is stored around the cell membrane. This protein build-up can reach a density which blocks cell permeability, so that there can no longer be adequate absorption of nutrients. Knowledgeable nutritional doctors, in fact, give their patients pancreatic enzymes in order to help digest the excess protein coating the cells, and thus allow sufficient nourishment to be utilized on the cellular level.

It is the quality of most meat products that one has to be concerned about because of the types of substances—synthetic growth hormones, antibiotics, rendered feed and other unnatural elements—which are used to make the animals marketable. Harmful residues may be left in the tissues. A doctor in Puerto Rico complained in a medical journal that she found girls were reaching puberty as early as eight and nine years of age.

She attributed it to the hormones in their meat. Studies have shown that these substances, when ingested into the human body, can be significant factors in the formation of degenerative diseases and cause resistance to antibiotics, a serious problem if a person needs them in a crisis.

Returning to the subject of foods that should be omitted from our diets, we certainly would include fried foods, because oils and fats that have been overly heated are difficult to digest and there have been hints that they may be carcinogenic. Overcooking is another aspect of food preparation that needs clarification. Keep in mind that enzymes, which are the catalysts to break down the food into its microcomponents, are destroyed at a temperature of about 115°F. and food cooked in water loses minerals. If the water is discarded, the minerals are lost.

Milk, despite industry claims, is not an adult food. It is intended by Nature to nourish infants. After about the age of two the body no longer produces the enzyme, lactase, essential for digesting milk. To take an artificial lactate enzyme which can be purchased in health food stores is to do something that the body contraindicates. Obviously, Nature has decided that milk is no longer useful for adults. There is no point in forcing the body to handle a food which it is not equipped to metabolize properly, and only burdens the eliminatory system with mucous and other wastes.

There is a great deal of concern about the possibility that the milk of nursing mothers might contain some chemicals from their own diets. Mothers should not make sudden dietary changes during their pregnancy or when they are nursing, because of the unexpected reactions that may result. As previously explained, the improved diet stimulates the release of toxins from the cells which make their way via the bloodstream to the fetus or to the infant through nursing. Hopefully, the mother has been on a good nutritional regime long before her pregnancy. In any event, we have to depend on the baby having a healthy elimination system, which Nature usually bestows on the very young. Mother's milk has been shown by government studies to be the ideal food for babies. It is the use of non-milk infant formulas that is particularly questionable. What sort of start is it for the newborn to be given man-formulated substances as its main nutritional element? Certainly, these products will sustain life, but do we know that they will encourage healthy growth to the degree that they should? And are we sure that the infant's organs will develop as normally as they should—or that he or she will not run into serious health problems 20, 30, or even 40 years later?

CHEMICAL ADDITIVES

There are hundreds of chemical additives in foods, including preservatives, colorings, flavorings, fixatives, emulsifiers, stabilizers and other synthetic materials that are legally permitted by the Food and Drug Administration (FDA). Agricultural chemicals are an additional hazard. Agricultural chemicals are now being added directly to seeds, instead of the soil, through genetic engineering. Although the FDA believes that the human body can tolerate small amounts of these substances, their standards do not take into account that some bodies accumulate toxic chemicals on a larger scale than others, so that the point of danger to health can arrive for one individual more readily than another. In addition, one must consider that the cumulative effect of many additives in combination with different foods over a long period of time, can bring some individuals more quickly to the point of toxic overload, and eventually to a biological breakdown.

Neither the manufacturers nor the government can establish a scientific yardstick to measure the amount of chemicalized materials the human system can tolerate. There is simply no way of knowing which individuals are going to be able to withstand the harmful effects for longer or lesser periods of time. This being so, anyone who is concerned with better nutrition should minimize their use of chemicalized food products and maximize those which are organically produced. Certainly, this is extremely important for individuals who have cancer or other serious ailments, and whose systems may already be burdened with waste, inadequate elimination and other dysfunctions.

Even fresh fruits and vegetables can be contaminated by residues of insecticides, pesticides, fungicides and other chemical substances that are routinely added to the soil. A story in the *Seattle Times* (July, 1997) reported on the routine, widespread use of fertilizers from sewage sludge that contain lead, arsenic, cadmium and radioactive wastes. In addition to contamination, the use of chemical fertilizers in high concentrations actually extracts from the soil essential elements needed to recreate Nature's balance for competent synergism. The purpose of chemical fertilizers, presumably, is to maintain good soil balance, but instead, the process of adding high-potency minerals upsets the essential balance of the soil.

There are still other ways in which foods are altered. It is reported, for instance, that some of the hybrid foods such as corn have less protein and other nutrients than natural corn. The new trend toward bio-engineered foods also tends to upset the normal synergism that exists in natural foods. The harm in using bio-engineered foods is arousing great controversy in scientific circles. A widely publicized study that created much alarm within a segment of the scientific community showed that milkweed pollen contaminated from genetically engineered corn caused the death of monarch butterflies. The negative effects that these alterations may have on the body have yet to be determined.

The fact that the human body tries to maintain health as best it can under these difficult circumstances, and makes every effort to eliminate toxic wastes in order to survive, makes it impossible to judge the cumulative harm that is being done to the human system, in that the effects are not immediately apparent but become evident only after years of abuse.

The public needs greater awareness of just what foods are unwholesome and should be limited in the cancer patient's diet. Our Food and Drug Administration simply doesn't have a proper yardstick to protect the American people from contaminated food products. It is up to an informed constituency to pressure the FDA to be *certain of safety* before granting approval of toxic chemicals. In the meantime, however, it is difficult to obtain and eat an ideal diet today. In order to have a balanced diet with all of the essential nutrients, we must tolerate some of the chemicalized materials. What we can do, however, is take a good deal of care when shopping to avoid chemically-treated food as much as possible. We can shop for organic produce and other organic goods that do not have chemical additives. But, when we have to use inorganic food in order to maintain a *balanced diet* (which is of paramount importance) we ought to do so with caution in the knowledge that they are far from ideal. If your diet as a whole is healthful enough, the better foods can help overcome the limited toxic substances that cannot be avoided, while still maintaining a balanced diet.

I am sometimes asked if there is some way to neutralize the herbicides and insecticides on fruits and vegetables. There is no scientific evidence that the cleansing processes used for this purpose actually do remove contaminants. Some suggested procedures are to soak the foods in a solution of apple cider vinegar and water. This is supposed to release some of the sprays from the foods—but we cannot be certain it does.

FOODS THAT BELONG IN THE DIET

I cannot emphasize enough that I am not making any suggestions for altering or improving the dietary regime that individuals are currently following. This is a process that can only be done safely and effectively by an experienced practitioner on an individualized basis. My intention is to provide general information on the fundamentals of better nutrition and to assist in making knowledgeable decisions. As I have indicated, this consists of eliminating foods which are in violation of sound nutrition and maintenance of health. The next step is to consider what Nature intended for the human organism to consume.

Raw Foods

Since man was not born with a method to cook food, we can consider cooking all our food was not Nature's intent. Nutritionists with years of experience have estimated that 70% of the foods we eat should be raw. Foods in their raw, whole form contain all the elements that the body should have—the minerals, vitamins and enzymes essential for the optimal utilization of other nutritional materials. Foods in their natural state are always nutritionally balanced. Where calcium is present, phosphorous, magnesium and other intrinsic elements will be present, too. Where you find potassium, you will find sodium as well. This is true not only with these minerals, but with a range of materials that Nature intends the human system to have in order for food to be properly digested and assimilated. In the raw state, it is precisely this synergistic combination of elements that makes for the best kind of metabolism.

Let me underline the fact that when you heat foods to the point where they are overcooked, there are losses not only in the valuable nutrients, but in the body's ability to metabolize these foods properly. When foods are heated to 115°F and above, the enzymes that are needed to metabolize them are no longer active. Of course, we have internal enzymes which are secreted by various glands of the body; but we also need the enzymes that naturally exist in foods for them to be processed more efficiently. Literally thousands of different enzymes are required to help break down proteins, fats, fibers, sugars, and starches into micronutrients that can be utilized for healthy cell production. There is no way for food to be absorbed into the bloodstream and be capable of producing healthy cells without the action of enzymes. Food that is overcooked to the degree that enzymes and other vital nutrients are depleted or destroyed is essentially food which cannot possibly nourish the cells as efficiently as raw foods.

It is true that the body can always take enough nourishment out of cooked food to survive, but it doesn't automatically maintain good health and high energy. Of course, not all the food has to be raw, but we do need an adequate amount of what we call "live food" to regain and maintain good health. As a matter of fact, many foods do not have to be heated to a temperature where the nutrients are destroyed. Corn, for example, is sweeter when it is uncooked. But if you are accustomed to having it hot, all you have to do is heat your water and put the corn in just long enough for it to become warm. Warming up your food is not the same as boiling it. Boiling alters some of the vital elements.

In addition to raw vegetables, the body also requires a sufficient amount of raw fruits. Unfortunately, in order to ensure that the fruits do not spoil before being marketed, and that they remain saleable as long as possible, too many of the fruits are picked in an unripened state. The result is that they never reach their maturity. In other words, the fruit does not develop all of the nutrients that are needed for properly nourishing the body.

For instance, fruits such as grapefruits, lemons and oranges are harvested entirely green, before they have reached their full sweetness. It is nearly impossible for most city dwellers to get tree-ripened citrus, which is actually so full of flavor and sweetness that it seems like a different food. In effect, many people have never tasted fruit in its natural condition. When citrus fruits are picked green and then chemically treated to achieve the orange and yellow color we are accustomed to seeing, their digestibility is weakened as well.

Anyone who is concerned with better nutrition should be aware that raw vegetables are the body's main nourishers; they contain a wide range of nutritional materials—each of which plays a specific role in the digestive and metabolic process. Though raw vegetables are preferable, vegetables may be steamed lightly without a loss in nutritional value. In their raw state, vegetables are basically alkaline foods, and are therefore important for acid/alkaline balance. By utilizing a broad range of vegetables—from beets and asparagus, carrots and zucchini, to lettuce and cucumbers—you can get the full range of the vitamin-enzyme-mineral and trace mineral factors that the body needs.

Fresh fruits are essential, too, since they serve as the body's cleansers, as well as contain valuable nutrients, especially glucose for energy. Contrary to what many people think, most fruits are alkaline or sub-acid, rather than acid. (The accompanying chart on page 92-93 will give you a better idea of which foods are acid and which are alkaline.) Fruits will be more alkaline when they are tree-ripened. As with vegetables, fruits should be varied in your daily diet as much as possible, preferably according to season, so that you can give your body the widest possible mix of nutrients.

Acid/Alkaline Balance

One of the major nutritional goals is to achieve proper acid/alkaline balance. It is important that the diet be more alkaline than acid. According to a number of research studies, this is the condition which is most conducive for the body's repair process.

There is a simple method for measuring pH (the symbol used as a measurement for acidity/alkalinity) in the urine which many practitioners suggest. One can buy nitrazine paper in any drug store. A half-inch or so of tape is dropped into a small amount of urine collected in a container. The tape turns to a color that is compared to a special chart on the package which gives the acid/alkaline numbers. A single urine test cannot give the total picture. The test ought to be repeated a number of times during the day, and over more than one day, to establish a pattern. Actually, the color will tend to fluctuate with the meals that are eaten. It never should be consistently too extreme on the acid side (which is called acidosis), or on the alkaline side (alkalosis). Either *extreme* is out of the normally healthy range.

Dr. William Howard Hay, author of the book, *How to Always Be Well*, whose own health broke down, decided during his long recovery that he would eat such things as were intended by Nature, taking them in their natural form and in quantities no greater than seemed necessary for his current needs. After three months, he began to recover from a heart condition that had been diagnosed incurable. He established a health clinic and devoted the remainder of his practice to treating diseases nutritionally, and found that his patients' health improved as a result of this natural healing regime.

According to Dr. Hay, one of the main causes of disease is acid formation due to the ingestion of too much meat. He followed Nature's dictate of using 80% alkaline-forming foods such as vegetables and fresh fruits, while only 20% of the food used was acid-forming (carbohydrates or protein). This combination of foods, plus a proper program for the elimina-

ACID-ALKALINE FOOD CHART

(Alkaline Foods appear in plain text; *Acidic Foods appear in italics*)

PROTEINS	*Cream Cheese*	Jerusalem	Swiss Chard
Beef	*Goat's Cheese*	Artichokes	Tomatoes
Chicken	*Goat's Whey*	Kohlrabi	Turnips
Duck	*Yellow Cheese*	Leeks	Watercress
Gelatin	FRESH	Lettuce	
Lamb	VEGETABLES	Lima Beans	FRESH
Turkey	Artichokes	Mushrooms	FRUITS
Venison	Asparagus	Okra	Apples
Crab	Beet Greens	Onions	Apricots
Flounder	Beets	Parsley	Blackberries
Haddock	Broccoli	Parsnips	Blueberries
Halibut	Brussel Spouts	Peas	Cantaloupe
Lobster	Cabbage	Peppers (Bell)	Cherries
Mackerel	Carrots	Pumpkin	Cranberries
Oysters	Cauliflower	Radishes	Currants
Pike	Celery	Rhubarb	Figs
Salmon	Corn	Rutabaga	Gooseberries
Shrimp	Cucumber	Sauerkraut	Grapefruit
Trout	Dandelion	Spinach	Grapes
Tuna	Greens	Squash	Honeydew
	Eggplant	(Summer	Melon
Eggs	Endive	and Winter)	Huckleberries
Cottage Cheese	Kale	String Beans	Kiwis
			Lemons

tion of waste build-up, was considered by Dr. Hay to be the prime way to achieve optimum health.

There has been an impression that the pH ought to be on the acid side in the 5.5 range. However, Dr. Hay and other healers have found that it should fluctuate from acid to alkaline, based on the food eaten. Since there was a controversy about acid/alkaline balance, FACT funded research, supervised by Flemming Rasmussen at McGill University in Canada, that verified a range closer to 7 was more conducive to maintaining and regaining health.

One of the basic principles that doctors such as Dr. Hay discovered

ACID-ALKALINE FOOD CHART

(Alkaline Foods appear in plain text; *Acidic Foods appear in italics*)

Limes	Apples	*Oats*	*Peanuts*
Oranges	Currants	*Popcorn*	*Pecans*
Papayas	Dates	*Rice (Brown)*	*Pine Nuts*
Peaches	Figs	*Whole Rye Flour*	*Walnuts*
Pears	Peaches	*Whole Wheat*	**LEGUMES AND**
Pineapples	Pears	*Flour*	**LENTILS***
Raspberries	Raisins	**FATS**	*Black Eyed Peas*
Strawberries	*Prunes*	Avocado	*Garbanzo Beans*
Tangerines		Ripe Olives	*Kidney Beans*
Watermelon	**FRESH NATURAL STARCHES**	*Butter*	*Lentils*
Youngberries	*Corn (Dried)*	*Cream*	*Lima Beans*
NATURAL SWEETS	*Coconuts*	*Olive Oil*	*Navy Beans*
	Chestnuts	*Peanut Oil*	*Split Peas*
Bananas	*Potatoes (Sweet)*	*Vegetable Oils*	*Pinto Beans*
Persimmons	*Potatoes (White)*	**NUTS**	
Honey	*Water Chestnuts*	Almonds	*Legumes and lentils are high in protein and carbohydrates. Dark beans are higher in protein and white beans are higher in starch.
Maple Sugar	*Yams*	Almond Butter	
Molasses		*Brazil Nuts*	
Sorghum	**DRY STARCHES**	*Cashews*	
Sugar (Raw)	*Barley (Unpolished)*	*Filberts*	
DRIED FRUITS	*Buckwheat*	*Hickory Nuts*	
Apricots	*Corn Meal*	*Peanut Butter*	

from long clinical experience and study is that healing is essentially the process of the body ridding itself of toxic materials. The body usually attempts to repair any biological dysfunctions when it is at rest in the evening or asleep; therefore, the most toxic time is the morning. Most people have been told repeatedly that a substantial breakfast is the best way to start the day. In many European health clinics the very opposite is the practice. They begin the early morning mostly with fruits which serve as cleansers, and then eat food on the alkaline side because this is one of the best ways to neutralize the overacidity from toxins and to stimulate the muscular activity of the intestines to eliminate wastes. After the period of morning toxicity is relieved, one can then start on the day's normal food intake.

The use of a potassium broth is an excellent procedure for arriving at proper alkalinity. In European clinics patterned after the Waerland healing method, a special alkaline broth called Excelsior or potassium broth is given to the patient as the first food item of the day. Prepared the evening before, the broth contains preferably organic unpeeled potatoes, onions, carrot, celery and other vegetables. The variety is unlimited. The vegetables are boiled for about a half hour in saltless water and then only the liquid is used, although the vegetables can be used in other ways. In the morning the broth is warmed up or served cold. This drink provides a rich supply of alkaline materials, and encourages the body to give up the harmful toxins that have gathered during the night. (This is a fine drink for people suffering from ulcers.)

A useful yardstick for establishing a balanced nutritional program for regaining health has been established by Dr. Bernard Jensen, former owner and director of the Hidden Valley Health Ranch in Escondido, California. The program meets the body's requirements by providing the entire range of elements needed to produce healthy cells, enhance immune vitality, maintain a clean internal environment, encourage waste elimination through good bowel function, and nourish and provide the energy necessary for healthful living.

Jensen's daily formula includes 6 vegetables, 2 fruits, 1 protein, 1 starch and whole, organic grains. I have added another ingredient—a fermented food, such as yogurt or naturally fermented vegetables. Fermented food provides the healthy intestinal flora that is a natural need of the colon. (See more about fermented food later in this chapter.)

Proteins

Proteins are the body's major cell-building materials. They should always be of high quality and uncontaminated from chemical additives, hormones or antibiotics. Vegetable proteins are available from nuts, sprouts, legumes (peas, beans, lentils) and avocados. Meat, fish, eggs, yogurt and cheese are a source of animal protein. Vegetables and grains contain smaller amounts of protein, but they are also good auxiliary sources.

Most people, although not all, need some kind of meat in their diet such as beef, lamb, fish, or fowl. There are some health practitioners that claim that man was designed by Nature to be a vegetarian. If this is so, the only thing I can conclude is that since the human system has a way of adapting to conditions, it has adapted to its environment in its natural effort to maintain life. It is therefore quite possible that the vast majority of individuals, having evolved from generations of meat-eating ancestors, require meat in their diet. The body, however, needs only a small quantity of meat protein and can't metabolize too much of it.

I have found that a low-protein diet is more appropriate for patients with cancer and other degenerative diseases than a no-protein or high-protein diet. Protein is one of the essential nutrients for cell production, but that doesn't necessarily mean that large quantities are better than adequate quantities. Too much protein puts a strain on the body's digestive capacity and may end up as excess storage material which interferes with cell nourishment and oxygenation. Too little protein, on the other hand, may lead to poor muscle tone, lack of energy, impaired healing ability, impaired cell production and less resistance to disease.

Dr. Robert Good, at the University of Minnesota, conducted an interesting experiment. He removed all protein from laboratory mice bred to produce tumors, and achieved tumor reduction. This result might leave the distinct impression that no protein is the universal answer to the cancer problem; however, he also discovered that when he extended the no-protein diet, the tumors regrew. We can conclude from this experiment that the body, by using up the stored protein, was able to maintain nutritional balance and achieve cancer cell reduction. But when protein deprivation continued after the body's protein reserves were depleted, the deficiency caused abnormal cell development again. This should teach us that the real answer to restoring health is *achieving nutritional balance.*

The recommended daily allowance of protein by the National Research Council is approximately 52 grams (about 2 ounces) for a male, with allowances for the man's size and degree of activity. The RDA for a non-nursing, non-pregnant female is approximately 46 grams (the equivalent of 1.6 ounces), with the same allowances. It is important to emphasize that these amounts are only approximations. These figures were confirmed by Jean Mayer, M.D., a highly regarded nutritionist and columnist in conventional medicine. This RDA is not too different from what had been advocated for many years earlier by practitioners in the natural health movement, as opposed to the widespread idea that an average of 120 grams of protein daily was the appropriate dietary requirement. Now, finally, in both conventional medicine and the natural health movement, there is agreement that less than half this amount is sufficient for good health.

The chart on page 98 indicates the protein values of various protein sources. It is being included for information only, and not as a guide for dietary changes. One should never undertake nutritional alterations—protein or otherwise—without competent help. A balanced nutritional regime depends on the patient's individual dietary requirements as a whole, and each doctor has his or her own way of balancing body chemistry.

As the chart indicates, there is a wide variety of protein sources available in our foods. The utilization of many different proteins will give the human system all of the essential amino acids necessary for building healthy cells.

Soy is a product which seems to have attracted something of a cult following as the perfect meat substitute or as a breast cancer preventive. I believe this is faddish and do not consider soy a good protein source as it is an enzyme inhibitor. It is unhealthy when it becomes the basis of a high-protein diet for individuals who want to change to vegetarianism. Since soy *inhibits enzymatic function*, it depletes food metabolism—*the very thing the cancer patient must avoid.*

Vegetable Juices

Metabolic programs often include vegetable juices which require the use of a vegetable juice extractor. This process separates the pulp from the liquid, and since most vegetables are 85% liquid, the juice will contain all the valuable nutritional elements. The discarded pulp is basically fiber. When you chew the vegetables in raw form, and break them down into pulp, mostly the liquid is absorbed. The pulp serves as roughage to clean the intestinal tract. With a vegetable juice extractor, one gets the combined benefits of many different vegetables in liquid form in far greater quantities than one could possibly have eaten in one meal. Of course, high fiber, such as pulp, is extremely important as roughage for waste elimination. It is usually acquired from salads, fruits and grains.

Sometimes, after being on a carrot juice regime for a while, one may note a yellow coloring in the skin. Dr. Norman Walker, who has written a number of excellent nutritional books including the most outstanding one on the subject of juicing, *Fresh Vegetable and Fruit Juices*, explains that the yellow coloring comes from the cleansing of the liver, which is stimulated by the juice itself. It will clear up when the liver is cleansed. He adds, "the carrot juice can no more cause a yellow skin color than a green vegetable juice can cause a green coloration." In Dr. Walker's book, different combinations of juices are taken to improve various body functions and to relieve some uncomfortable symptoms. When beets are taken in small quantities, for example, they are excellent for cleansing the bowels and the lymphatic system. They can also stimulate a liquefied bowel movement, and cause red color to appear in the urine. That can be disconcerting to those who do not know in advance that it can happen. Cabbage juice which contains vitamin K (the clotting vitamin) is considered appropriate for bleeding ulcers and colitis. These are only a few of the examples you'll find in Walker's book.

As with all other dietary improvements, juicing may induce the body to unexpected healing reactions. In my experience, many people may take vegetable juice—and this is something that Dr. Walker writes about—and feel more gassy than they have ever felt before and make the assumption that they are allergic. This does not occur because the juice is harmful or is generating the gas. It is the result of putrefied material being dislodged from storage by the action of the juice. As these putrefied wastes pass through the intestines, they produce uncomfortable symptoms. Eventually, this gassy feeling will wear off and drinking the same identical juice will no longer cause this reaction. Indeed, this is why practitioners who place their patients on vegetable juices will invariably advise detoxification procedures first. This is to help the body get rid of the wastes that are being dislodged from storage by the cleansing action of the abundant juice intake.

Grains

Grains are complex carbohydrates which contain a rich source of vital nutrients. Grains are actually the seeds of various plants and in whole form are one of the most beneficial foods available. They contain all the elements needed to produce new life (plants) and new seeds. Because they reproduce, they are an unusual source of natural balanced hormones. Milling or processing grains deprives them of much of their nutritional value. The grain should be in whole form, including the germ (the growing part of the seed); the large endosperm (mostly starches, with a small amount of proteins, minerals and vitamins); and the bran covering (which is largely cellulose, with traces of minerals, vitamins and proteins). When

PROTEIN VALUES IN WHOLE FOOD

	Approx. Grams		Approx. Grams
NUTS (2 OUNCES)		1 cup of milk	9
almonds	10	1 ounce of meat	7
Brazil nuts	8	1 egg	6
cashews	9		
filberts	7	1 tbsp peanut butter	4
pecans	5	1 slice of whole wheat	
walnuts	8	bread	3
LEGUMES (2 OUNCES)		1 cup of spinach	5
peanuts	16	1 medium baked potato	3
dried peas	15	1 cup of yogurt	8
dried chickpeas	11	3½ ounces of most	
dried lima beans	4.5	cooked vegetables	2–4
GRAINS (2 OUNCES)		1 ounce of cheese	7
barley	5	1 medium avocado	5
millet	5	6 ounces of fish	41
brown rice	4		
bran	8		
rice polish	7	Some of the figures shown	
rye	7	above were computed from	
wheat	8	*Composition of Foods* by Hermitage	
raw wheat germ	16	Press and from an article by	
		Dr. Jean Mayer.	

the whole grain is eaten intact, it provides the body with all of these nutrients, in synergistic balance as Nature intended.

The flavor of the whole grain is much better than that of the processed forms. Most people have become accustomed to the bland taste of the cereal they usually purchase in the supermarket, even though there is actually little difference in taste and texture between most of these processed cereals. We like to refer to the whole grains as live food because its valuable vitamins, minerals and enzymes have not been altered or killed by heat or processing. In fact, it has been found that whole grains from ancient Egyptian tombs—thousands of years old—sprouted when planted!

You certainly could not do this with a processed grain product that has been put through hot rollers, or deprived of its bran or germ, and joined with preservatives to lengthen its storage time and shelf-life.

I feel that we must be careful when we take parts of a food rather than the whole. Even using the bran without the "meat" is not advisable. It corrupts the natural synergism of the grain. Nature prepared food in its entirety, and for the most part, this is the way it should be eaten. The natural combination of vitamins, minerals and enzymes is what makes food synergistically sound and competently metabolized.

There are many different grains from which to choose: rye, oats, wheat, barley, brown rice, millet, couscous, buckwheat (kasha), corn, as well as many more. There is an excellent method of preparing the grain with the use of a Thermos. It is even simpler and certainly healthier than the quick-cooking grains you buy at the supermarket and, more importantly, it will retain the full flavor, natural enzymes and living nutrients of the grains.

Thermos-cooked cereal is the most wholesome way of preserving the precious elements to the optimum degree possible. The method originated at the Waerland Clinics in Europe and was adapted to the Thermos by Dr. Bernard Jensen. All that is necessary is a wide-mouth Thermos and the whole grains that the individual prefers. Rye, barley and oats do not need to be ground before the thermos-cooking process, but the others will not soften adequately if not ground beforehand in an ordinary blender or a seed mill. The grains can be used singly or in combination for different tastes. It is interesting to experiment to achieve various flavors that are satisfying.

To prepare the cereal, put three tablespoons of the grain in the thermos and add one cup of hot water as the average portion. If more or less is desired, use a ratio of ⅓ cup of water to 1 tablespoon of cereal. Let stand overnight or for about eight hours. The result will be the equivalent of prepared cereal without the loss of its nutritional value or destruction of valuable enzymes. Some people prefer to use the cereal in its whole form as it comes from the thermos. Others like to grind it in a blender for a soft, more familiar consistency. If the cereal needs to be rewarmed, put it in a bowl and warm it over hot water. This is similar to using a double boiler except that a pot and a bowl are used. Do not overheat!

To give the cereal additional flavor, add honey, maple syrup, bananas or other fresh fruit. If raisins or dates are used, they can be soaked overnight in the thermos with the grains. Or if the raisins or dates are soaked separately, add the liquid to the cereal as a good sweetener. Cream can be used in small quantities, because it is a different product than milk. It is a fat and doesn't require lactase enzymes to be metabolized.

Nut milk is another excellent food that can be added to the cereal. Almond milk is delicious, very alkaline, high in protein, and easy to assimilate and absorb. It can be made by soaking almonds overnight in distilled water or apple or pineapple juice. Three ounces of the soaked nuts are put into five ounces of liquid and blended for two to two and one half minutes in a liquefier. In addition to cereal, nut milk goes well with any kind of fruit, juice or vegetable juice, and is also a good alkaline drink. Other nuts or seeds such as sesame, sunflower, or walnuts can be substituted for almonds but they are not alkaline. Sesame seeds are an exceptionally good source of calcium. Besides grains, other quality carbohydrates include potatoes (both white and sweet), winter squash and beans of all kinds— lima, navy, chickpeas, red kidney, etc. Potatoes and winter squash are best when baked or steamed, and of course the beans have to be cooked in order to be utilized. When the beans are soaked in advance, they cook more quickly and retain more of their nutrients.

Oils and Fats

Oils and fats provide the body with fatty acid which is an essential part of the diet. The body needs these fatty acids for energy, proper vitamin utilization, protecting the organs and coating the nerves, and other functions.

Although excessive amounts of fat in the diet are burdensome for the liver to metabolize, the body does require a certain amount of fatty acid. One should take care, however, not to cook foods in oil. Heated oil for frying has been found to be carcinogenic in laboratory animals. The nature of oil changes when heated, so that the body cannot deal with it comfortably. Oils are present in nuts, grains, avocado and in other vegetables as well. Fatty acids are also found in butter, cream, eggs and flesh foods.

One does not have to discard all of the fatty acids, or heap oil on all foods. On salads, for example, a little cold-pressed oil from good raw sources is quite acceptable. Lemon and herbal seasonings added make an excellent salad dressing. Yogurt, avocado, tahini or other nut butters also make good salad dressing foundations. It is also possible to make your own healthful mayonnaise by using eggs, oil, lemon and whatever flavorings you like. If people are accustomed to and want salad dressings, there are many wholesome ingredients to choose from. It goes without saying that no hydrogenated fat, margarines or lard should be used, as they burden the liver.

Sprouts

Sprouts are considered one of the finest all-around sources of vitamins, minerals and enzymes, as well as many other vital nutrients. They are actually living foods which can be grown at home. (Today many supermarkets carry a variety of sprouts.) Almost any seed, grain or legume can be sprouted, including alfalfa, rye, radish, and so forth. A simple method for growing sprouts is as follows: Use a 1-quart wide-mouth jar and a piece of cheesecloth or mesh fastened with a rubber band as a cover. Depending on which you prefer, put either 2 tablespoons of alfalfa seeds; or 2 tablespoons of fenugreek; or $\frac{1}{4}$ cup lentils or $\frac{1}{4}$ cup mung beans into the jar. (You can also use these seeds in various combinations.) Soak the seeds for about 15 hours then drain the water. Afterwards rinse and drain well twice daily for about 3 to 5 days. Simply place underneath the faucet and rinse morning and evening. These seeds grow abundantly in a few days. When the seeds sprout, put them in a sunny place for photosynthesis so that the leaves turn green. Sprouts are delicious in salads, soups, when eaten plain, or added to any vegetable, egg or fish dish for flavor and nourishment.

Sprouts contain all the nutrients the plant needs for life and growth. They are storehouses of carbohydrates, protein, vitamins, minerals, oil and natural sugars, in their most assimilable form for the cells of the human body. They are not only tasty and easy to grow, but low in cost.

Fermented Foods

Fermented food is always considered appropriate, as part of a nutritional regime, in order to supply the intestinal flora necessary for good digestion and elimination. Preservatives added to processed foods destroy the healthy bacteria (flora). When the colon is functioning well, it harbors what are often called "friendly intestinal flora." Excellent ferments can be obtained by using products derived from soured milk such as yogurt, clabbered milk or kefir. Rejuvelac is a non-dairy fermented product developed by Ann Wigmore at the Hippocrates Health Center. It is made by soaking wheat berries in water until they sour (about 24 to 36 or more hours). The liquid has a mildly tart flavor and is very refreshing, especially as a cool drink in the summertime. The berries can be reused up to 3 times. Fermented products are considered predigested; that is, the bacteria starts the digestive process making nutrients more available to the body. One can also use sauerkraut, pickles or other vegetables if they are naturally fermented without vinegar or salt. There are some companies that produce lactic acid juices which are also suitable as a fermented food to complete the dietary essentials.

To prepare yogurt, open the top of a carton of certified raw milk. Without removing the milk from the carton, thoroughly mix in three tablespoons of previously-made yogurt or a packet of yogurt culture as a starter. Place some loose covering on top and leave in a warm place for 24 hours or until the contents have thickened. Or pour the contents into individual containers. Refrigerate before serving. Your first batch of yogurt will be slightly liquid; subsequent batches will be thicker.

Glucose

The body's cells require glucose for energy, but one has to be certain that the source of glucose is obtained from natural sources, such as fruit, starches, raw honey or a good maple syrup (processed without formaldehyde).

Natural sugar is brown and sticky and has lots of vitamins and minerals, but these have been processed out to provide a more manageable product. If you use refined sugar, either in the granulated form or in any of the myriad foods in which it appears, it does not have the natural nutrients that the body needs to be metabolized properly. An excess of refined sugar can rob the body of vitamins essential for metabolizing carbohydrates, exhaust the pancreas, and in addition become addictive. (Americans consume an average of more than 120 pounds of sugar annually.) It is therefore essential that only healthful sources of glucose are part of the diet—fruit, honey, raw sugar, etc.

Food Supplements

Food supplements are materials in concentrated form that can be added to the diet when there is a specific deficiency of enzymes, vitamins, minerals or other nutrients. They need to be of excellent quality and individualized for the patient. Supplements should not be taken indiscriminately. The key to restoring health is to achieve balance; imbalance can be created from excessive use of supplements.

We need to understand the nature of supplements—the hazards as well as the usefulness. Some people have, for many years, been under the impression that there would be no harm in taking all kinds of supplementary material in any dosage. We have become far more sophisticated and now know that the body can become seriously imbalanced if it is given more supplements than it requires; overdoses disrupt body chemistry and deplete the system of other elements that are needed to complement a fragmented supplement.

Another factor that is not well enough understood is that supplements were produced originally from food substances. These food materials were dehydrated by a special process and made into tablets. Because they were biologically-sound materials that contained all the vital nutrients, the supplements were then synergistically utilizable.

Today, there are only a few companies which are still making supplements of that quality. A great deal of the material now available is synthetic, so the supplements are incomplete or fragmented. Even though we hear people say, "I buy it in my health food store and the label says all-natural," this does not mean that the product is without coloring, synthetic additions or preservatives. For the most part, potency is usually achieved by using synthetic additives. For example, many health food stores carry "natural" vitamin C with rose hips, usually meaning the product contains a few mgs of rose hips and the rest is processed or factory-produced ascorbic acid.

In addition, many companies add U.S. certified colors, which should be avoided, and preservatives to assure a long shelf-life. In view of these deviations from high standards that we ought to expect, the process by which each company manufactures its products should be carefully determined. Inferior quality may jeopardize the healing process.

People sometimes take megadoses of vitamins, either on their own or with amateur advice, in the belief that it can help prevent or overcome cancer and other serious health conditions. Actually, a vitamin deficiency can be created due to the intake of the wrong type of supplements, instead of too little. Dr. Royal Lee, one of the pioneers in the development of and interest in vitamins, became quite alarmed about the improper use of vitamin supplements and the poor standards used in manufacturing them. He alerted people to bear in mind the frequency with which vitamin supplements are ordinarily taken (three times a day). Because of this, he warned, it is critically important for an individual to know the kinds of supplementary materials he or she is ingesting, and the quantity likely to produce the desired results. Without this knowledge, one cannot be sure that the quantity and quality are not an overdose likely to aggravate the problem instead of alleviating it.

In an article entitled, "The Fallacy of High Potency in Vitamin Dosage," Dr. Lee noted that "there is ample proof that many vitamins may cause, in excess quantities, the same symptoms that are caused by their deficiency. Vitamin B1 in small dosage can cure herpes zoster; large doses can cause herpes zoster." Explaining that vitamin E affects calcium balance, he pointed out that an overdose violates the essential synergism, leaving the body unable to metabolize the very vitamins that are being used. Dr. Lee also writes about the acute deficiency conditions that can be caused by overdoses of vitamins D, E and K.

A belief that has pervaded the health movement is that virtually all of the foods today are depleted because of poor soil; therefore, we all need supplementation. That is not accurate. Some people's bodies are depleted, others are not. We can include a wide range of foods in our diets, so that even though a deficiency may exist in one food, it may be sufficient in other foods. Therefore, we do not necessarily have to be suffering from nutritional deficiencies. Sometimes the vitamins and minerals are available but the body is not metabolizing them. In that instance, enzymes are needed to metabolize the available vitamins and minerals, instead of assuming there is a deficiency and resorting to megadoses.

Let me emphasize, if you take supplements—which are largely made of synthetic chemicals—the body will have to use its own stored minerals, vitamins and enzymes in order to reconstitute the missing ingredients into a natural complex for absorption. Eventually, the overdrawing of these supplements will seriously deplete the body of the missing essential elements and cause the deficiency that one is trying to overcome.

GUIDELINES FOR FOOD PREPARATION AND EATING

What kinds of utensils should be used in food preparation? Studies have shown that aluminum—a highly toxic metal—can seep into the food. If you look carefully at an aluminum utensil that has been used for a while, you will find that it is pitted. What this indicates is that the acid in the food tends to leach small but harmful quantities of aluminum into the food.

FOOD FOR THOUGHT

■ Biorepair systems automatically enhance the immune system if the program is effective and the patient's body is capable of responding. Care must be taken to avoid rejection when patients have had implants of plastic or metal. A revitalized immune system will seek out foreign material and attempt to reject it. Foreign material may include: clips used in surgery, plastic stents, artificial heart valves, breast implants, dental implants, joint replacements, lens replacements, plastic mesh used for hernia repair, ear prosthesis, etc.

■ Canola oil is actually rape seed genetically engineered to lessen the level of toxic erucic acid. Unaltered rape seed oil is only used as an industrial oil because erucic acid is highly toxic. Through genetic engineering the erucic acid was lessened, but not eliminated. Cancer patients should avoid products that contain canola oil.

■ Avoid soy products in spite of the promotion of soy as an effective substance to prevent breast cancer. The final answer is not yet in. Soy is an enzyme inhibitor. Enzyme inhibition would obstruct the metabolism of nutritional elements which are essential for healthy cell production.

■ Vegetarianism is considered a healthful diet by some practitioners and people against the slaughter of animals for ethical reasons. It seems to have great appeal for young people who want to maintain their health. Unfortunately, they may be the least likely candidates for vegetarianism. For most people, flesh protein is essential for a balanced diet and needed for healthy cell production. There may have been a time when humans were vegetarians, but this may have changed because the body adapted to the meat eating diet of our ancestors.

■ Women of child-bearing age, who are planning to conceive, should avoid changing their diet at least a year before conception to allow the body sufficient time to detoxify. If their body is toxic, the improved diet will attempt to "clean house." The process causes the release of toxins from storage into the bloodstream. This will then be fed to the uterus through the placenta and can cause complications. This caution also applies to nursing the infant.

Teflon utensils, because they give off gasses at high heat, should be avoided. It is preferable to use cooking utensils that do not contaminate the food—such as, Corningware, glass, stainless steel, enamel, and iron pots that have been seasoned so they do not rust.

Eating should be an occasion for enjoying your food and not rushing through the meal. Eat slowly, and savor every bit of food and sip of liquid, whether it is water, herb teas, or other beverages. It is well said that vegetable juices ought to be eaten slowly and salivated, like solid foods. And solid foods, of course, ought to be chewed well, until they are liquefied in your mouth, because the digestive process starts in the mouth. As Dr. Karl Aly, retired director of a 90-bed health clinic in Sweden, put it, "Chew your liquids and drink your solids." Ptyalin, one of the digestive enzymes, is present in the mouth just for this purpose. When you gulp down big chunks of food, it bypasses the enzymatic function of the ptyalin and places a burden on the digestive juices in the stomach.

Food should never be eaten when one is under stress. If you come home tired, wait until the tiredness subsides. Relax and try to release all of your tensions before you start your meal. Extreme stress will alter the whole metabolic process by triggering changes in the digestive secretions—either too much or too little. As a result, foods will not be broken down to the microscopic form in which they are most readily accessible to the cells.

We cannot dictate to our bodies what our eating pattern should be. Unfortunately, because of our business and work habits, we are ordinarily required to eat three meals a day at stated times—breakfast in the morning, lunch at noon and dinner in the evening. Food should be eaten as nature intends—only when we are hungry, whether it is two, four or six times a day. Let your appetite be your guide, not your clock. And remember, unlike highly-seasoned, processed or otherwise chemicalized products, wholesome foods have subtle flavors and taste delicious. This becomes more apparent as we come to appreciate them.

In nutrition, as elsewhere, it is important for individuals to listen to what their bodies are telling them. We are created with all sorts of autonomic reactions, which are Nature's way of communicating to our conscious minds what is taking place internally. If you experience pain, or any other distressing symptom, there is a good reason to heed the signal. If you feel nauseous or without an appetite, it is actually a message from your body telling you not to eat—that it is not in a position to metabolize the foods you will ingest.

Dr. Edwin Flatto expressed this idea very aptly. "Don't put any more coals in the furnace when you have a headache, or no appetite," he noted, "it's the stomach telling the brain not to eat any food because the body has enough waste to get rid of."

I should like my readers to be aware that the nutritional concepts I have been discussing are applicable to all individuals—whatever their state of health. The difference is, however, that there are special considerations in the case of the cancer patient. Even in the early stages of cancer, the patient's biological impairments or breakdowns are undoubtedly more severe. Whatever corrections need to be made, nutritional or otherwise, must be done more carefully in every aspect of their health.

Like all biological repairs, nutritional changes provoke all kinds of symptoms. Relying on nutrition as a therapy for helping to repair a biological dysfunction goes beyond a sound diet. Even if you eat the most healthful, wonderful foods, you can create problems if you throw your body chemistry out of balance by taking an excess of synthetic supplements, letting your wastes build up, or neglecting any other health problem. And let us not neglect the state of our emotions and the havoc it can play on metabolic secretions.

I hope that reading this material will provide a good background of just how complex and potent nutrition can be. It will be up to the practitioner to plan your dietary regime on the basis of his or her knowledge and experience. To a large extent, however, your own intelligence in nutritional matters—and about the process of biological repair as a whole—will help you carry out this metabolic program more effectively. Not only should the patient want to participate actively in his or her healing process, but most doctors will do their best to encourage this partnership.

6. Detoxification: Prerequisite for Repair

*The more nourishment you give to a person who
has not been purged, the more harm you do.*
—HIPPOCRATES

As I have noted earlier, detoxification is one of the most critically important aspects of a health restoration program—yet it is an area that causes the greatest misunderstanding, controversy and confusion among patients and professionals who are using biological repair techniques. To begin with, what is toxicity? Exactly what is meant by detoxifying the human system? Why is this life-process essential for preventing diseases and repairing biological dysfunctions? What are some of the procedures that competent practitioners utilize to help the body rid itself of toxins? These are among the questions which I want to deal with in some depth in the following pages.

THE CONCEPT OF TOXICITY

All of us, without exception, are exposed to food additives, drugs, cosmetics, household chemicals, environmental pollutants and other toxic substances from the day we are born. If the interrelated system of eliminatory organs is not operating as efficiently as it ought to, the body is not going to be able to overcome the harmful effects of this toxic overload. Of course, the effects of these accumulated wastes and the ability to eliminate them, differ from individual to individual. When people are exposed to the same conditions, as for example workers in a chemical factory, some will get sick and others will not. One of the reasons for this is that some human systems

have a greater degree of host resistance, and can discard wastes more efficiently. Host resistance can depend on factors such as endowment with a
stronger constitution or following a healthier lifestyle—physically, mentally, nutritionally and environmentally.

In any event, poor waste elimination will be reflected in a colon that is
sluggish with poor muscle tone. Or in a liver that is not working at normal
capacity; or there may be other biological impairments of the various eliminatory organs. The result will be storage of the backed-up wastes in the tissues and glands.

The idea that excessive accumulations of toxins within the human
body can precipitate any number of chronic, degenerative diseases has
been the basis of healing for many years by physicians practicing natural
healing. It remained a theory, however, until the early part of this century,
when other doctors, practitioners and scientists validated the concept
independently of one another through considerable research and clinic
experience.

One of them, a physician, J.H. Tilden, M.D., wrote a book called
Toxemia Explained in which he described toxemia as a condition which
occurs when a high concentration of poisons accumulates in the cells, tissues, lymphatics and blood to the extent that they impede normal body
functions, including the efficiency of the eliminatory organs. As the chemicals, food additives and other toxins to which we are exposed in our daily
lives accumulate, the cycle continues, intensifying the whole destructive
process. According to Dr. Tilden, it is this high level of poisons within the
body's tissues that is responsible for weakening the body's ability to function efficiently. At a level at which the body can no longer cope, the toxins
lead to manifestations of disease—from the degeneration of the joints in
arthritis, through gastrointestinal and glandular problems, to metabolic
breakdowns, nerve disorders and cancer.

Dr. Tilden states that one needs to be convinced that toxic wastes are
among the major precipitating factors in all diseases, and that lowering
the concentration of body wastes to a non-toxic level is one of the most
fundamental aspects of the healing process. The research and clinical
experience of many physicians and health practitioners, mostly in Europe
but increasingly in the United States, has confirmed in many respects the
overall validity of the theory that toxicity plays a key role in the development of degenerative conditions.

Years ago, the subject of alimentary toxemia was discussed in London before the Royal Society of Medicine by 57 of Great Britain's leading physicians. Among the speakers were distinguished surgeons, physicians and specialists in various branches of medicine. Some of them pointed out that a combination of different chemicals and other poisonous materials within the colon, even in small quantities, can produce the most profound consequences. This concept is still valid today.

The claim was not made that toxins were the only cause of the symptoms of disease. Some of the doctors, however, did point out that putrefied waste stored in the colon for too long was a principal factor in the development of diseases ranging from multiple sclerosis, chronic fatigue syndrome, to nerve disorders and other breakdowns. Dr. W. Bezley noted that, "there are few phases of cardiovascular trouble with which a disorder of some part of the alimentary tract is not actively associated." Another physician stated that "an infinitesimal amount of poison may suffice to cause skin eruption." Others related excessive levels of toxicity to headaches, irritation of the nervous system, and diseases of the genitourinary organs.

I should make it clear that these findings are not merely theories but are the result of demonstrations in actual practice among many physicians who use biologically-sound healing methods. This array of evidence—as well as the clinical experiences of many practitioners—makes it difficult to ignore the implications of the relationship between toxicity and most diseases. On the contrary, the medical establishment is today beginning to be more receptive to the concept that the body accumulates toxins that do not belong in the human system—food additives, drugs, carcinogens, dead cells from excessive x-ray dosages—until their effect becomes cumulatively destructive. Increasingly, conventional doctors, as well as practitioners who support biological concepts of healing, are agreeing that cancer may be caused by accumulations of chemicals from the food supply. The World Health Organization estimates that more than 85% of cancers are environmentally induced; that means from food, air, water and the work place. A number of chemical food additives have been shown to be cancer-triggering substances. Although many food additives are suspected of being cancer-linked, so few are tested for carcinogenicity over a long period of time that it is impossible to know the total number.

Following is an example of a chemical effect on the human system based on the research of Dr. Ben Finegold, M.D. When his work was first published, it caused the typical controversy and was negated by resources representing the chemical industry—not an unusual response. Whenever privately-funded research jeopardizes an industry's welfare, their response is to fund research which negates the original conclusion. Nevertheless, I feel strongly that Dr. Finegold's studies cannot be ignored.

He studied the effect of food additives on hyperactive children who are restless in school, have trouble concentrating and are chronically misbehaving. He rightly concluded that the condition was generated by chemical additives put in foods to which the children reacted. I can assume that the chemicals irritated their nervous system. As part of the research study, the children were put on a good diet of carefully selected food without chemical additives. Their behavior became normal, but when they were once again given food with additives—substances that are alien to the human system—they again exhibited hyperkinetic symptoms. It took *three days* before elimination of the toxicity from the additives was completed and the body was finally able to relax and return to normal. It is obvious from these studies that many dangerous substances are not easily eliminated from the body, and as long as they remain in the human system, the abnormal conditions caused by the toxins will continue to manifest in troubling symptoms.

We cannot wait for our government agencies to officially determine what is carcinogenic. Their current position is that if it hasn't been proven harmful it is considered safe. (The official term is GRAS—Generally Recognized As Safe.) The position should be the very opposite; if it hasn't been proven safe, it should not be approved for human use. There are many things that have been approved by the FDA, which after extended use on the human population, had to be removed from the approved list because they were found to be hazardous even to the point of causing death. We have to use good judgement to evaluate clinical evidence— feedback from patients and our own physiology in order not to be one of the guinea pigs that failed.

Certainly, conventional medicine utilizes treatments and drugs (some of which are ineffective or even harmful) without waiting for the ultimate scientific proof by evaluating or conducting the research over an extended period of time. I do not mean to suggest that scientific validation of medical practices is not necessary. On the contrary, in my position I am extremely careful to withhold support from any alternative therapy or resource until it has proven its safety and effectiveness in many clinical experiences *over an extended period of time.* Time is an extremely important factor, especially relative to cancer, in evaluating a new drug or treatment modality. I feel that our government agencies are not allowing adequate time before determining safety.

The list of toxic substances—whether they are in our food, air, water, or on the job—keeps growing at an alarming rate. In the light of this evidence, it seems to me that it should not be too great a leap to conclude that toxins of all kinds that find their way into the body are among the most significant factors in the production of degenerative diseases. I sincerely believe that it is only a matter of time before the medical and scientific community accepts, to a greater degree, the concept that accumulated toxins play a devastating role in causing the major biological breakdowns that underlie cancer; and conversely, a system of biological repair that includes methods of ridding the body of these toxins is an essential aspect of any sound biological cancer treatment.

THE NEED FOR DETOXIFICATION

If one is going to utilize biological therapies to reverse a state of ill health, it is imperative to assist the body in the removal of toxins to avoid the discomfort that occurs when the bloodstream is overloaded, albeit temporarily. Some form of detoxification should be followed by the patient so that the cells, tissues and organs can be relieved and thereby regain normal function. All of my investigations, discussions with clinicians from European clinics and elsewhere, and my experience and feedback with patients leads to this conclusion. It is hard to imagine a situation where a patient with cancer or other degenerative disease can make real progress toward full recovery, in a fundamental and long-range sense, without including procedures for eliminating the stored body wastes.

Poor elimination of toxins will have a destructive effect on the immune system, which is known to play an active role in preventing and fighting cancer. The immune mechanism, to a large degree, depends on the health of the elimination system. Poor elimination of toxins puts a strain on the immune system. Its job is to seek out any foreign substances and process them for elimination—and cancer cells are regarded as foreign substances by the immune system. Therefore, when there is a sluggishness in the elimination of toxins, their presence may eventually exhaust or overload the immune system's effort to "clean house," and cause a weakening in the body's defenses against cancer.

Every effort will have to be made by the patient to attack and eliminate this backup of waste products. Unless ways of ridding the body of toxic materials is included in a program, the patient is going to be left with the same biological impairment that originally led to the disease. Even if the tumor is totally removed, the cause of the body's dysfunction will remain. In essence, this accounts for the situation where traditional treatment—whether it be surgery, chemotherapy or radiation—can bring about only a temporary respite from the cancer, as those treatments have not dealt with the cause.

It's worth repeating that the body's elimination system can break down for a number of reasons: hereditary weaknesses, poor nutrition, structural interferences with the nerves that instruct the organs to function normally, prolonged exposure to carcinogens, and so forth. Usually, because of one or a combination of these factors, organs may become dysfunctional to the point where they are too exhausted to do their work. This may be temporary or prolonged.

Let's take the liver as an example; one of its many jobs is to cleanse the bloodstream. Toxins removed by the liver are dumped into the intestines through the bile duct, eventually to be eliminated at the anal area. Competent colon function is essential so that the toxins are not reabsorbed through the portal vein and recirculated again and again, thus exhausting the liver, the master organ. If the lungs can no longer do their job, the patient won't have sufficient oxygen/waste exchange. If the skin is not perspiring sufficiently, or is hampered from performing its function by antiperspirants that block the elimination of wastes through the underarm pores, it will allow toxins to accumulate in the bloodstream. The kidneys, too, can be exhausted to the degree that they cannot cleanse the urine efficiently, leaving a dangerous accumulation of toxins in the body. Since these waste materials, which were instrumental in producing the state of ill health, are not being sufficiently eliminated due to weakened organ function, special techniques have to be utilized to assist the body in cleansing the internal environment.

The Colon and Elimination

The colon and kidneys are the prime organs of elimination. The colon needs a great deal of attention. It can become encrusted with dried fecal matter that hampers the action of the musculature, or pocketed with putrefied material that constantly feeds toxicity back into the bloodstream.

It is hard to convey by words alone the accumulated damage that can occur to the colon as a result of chronically ingesting poor quality fiberless food, lack of exercise, or sluggish peristalsis—the body's process of moving food through the digestive tract. Dr. Harvey W. Kellogg, a noted surgeon, indicated in the early part of the last century just how widespread these conditions were when he wrote: "Of the 22,000 operations I personally performed, I never found a single normal colon, and of the 100,000 that were performed under my jurisdiction, not over 6% were healthy."

When the wastes move slowly through a sluggish and distorted colon on their way to elimination at the anus, the foods begin to putrefy. Let me remind you that the human colon is at least five to six feet long, and that is a long distance for the wastes to move from the time they enter at the ileocecal valve (where the small intestine leads into the colon). And when there are convolutions, twists, bulges and extremely narrow areas in the colon because of poor muscle tone, these distortions can further impede the movement of wastes. Eventually, unless removed from the body, the accumulated wastes can contribute to a wide range of organ weaknesses and the biological breakdowns I have described. If the wastes remain there too long, they may cause an inflammatory condition. Stress, too, can restrict the colon's normal function of eliminating waste. These conditions can be prevented and corrected if the colon is kept clean.

The pioneering work of Sir William Arbuthnot Lane, M.D., noted physician and surgeon to the royal family of England at the beginning of the 20th century, provides significant evidence of what waste materials remaining in the colon can do. After operating on a patient with rheumatoid arthritis to remove an inflamed piece of colon, he amazingly discovered that the young man recovered from his severe arthritic condition and was able to give up the wheelchair to which he was restricted. This phenomenon motivated Dr. Lane to research the situation carefully. Ultimately, he found that different parts of the colon related through nerves to various organs. By excising the offending piece of colon, he was able to alleviate chronic disease conditions. Dr. Lane taught this surgical procedure to his students, and followed it in his own practice. He finally concluded that perhaps it was unnecessary to do colon surgery at all; merely removing the wastes which were causing the inflammation or other problems in the colon was the wiser way to handle the problem. Toward this end, he proposed that colon cleansing was a preferable procedure, not only to correct colon complications, but to prevent them. "I do not believe it is possible," he wrote, "for rheumatoid arthritis to obtain a foothold except in the presence of intestinal stasis." It may be remembered that at one time it was popular to take mineral oil to clean the colon; this was based on a suggestion of Dr. Lane.

I find it particularly unfortunate that the medical establishment, by and large, has long felt that infrequent bowel movements can be a normal pattern for some individuals. Of course, life will go on, sometimes even without apparent ill effects, but that does not mean that a disease condition will not develop in the future. Constipation is a sluggish movement in the bowels. It indicates that the colon musculature has lost its tone, and with this, the ability to move the feces to the rectum as efficiently as it should.

Very often, I have heard people say, "I move my bowels every day; I don't need any help." The truth is, however, that in many people the colon is not doing the job of propelling the feces by means of peristalsis from the entrance valve of the colon to the anus. Even though individuals may be moving their bowels daily, the process of elimination is being accomplished solely because the waste entering the colon is pushing the previous day's waste forward until it reaches the rectum. Meal after meal pushes the waste along. Sometimes the waste eliminated in this fashion may be two, three, four days old, or even older. This transit time is too long, giving the waste time to putrefy and harden.

Sometimes the passageway can become quite narrow because of a thick, hard accumulation of fecal matter on the intestinal wall. Or one can have bulges in the colon which become filled with waste, the weight of which stretches the colon, creating an additional narrowing from the weight on other areas. A constipated colon with narrowed areas restricts the normal movement of waste.

There is no way to know for certain if this is happening. But when it does, experienced practitioners will advise the individual as to the best means to clean the colon, such as colon irrigation. Once the cement-like material is removed, the muscles will be given a chance to repair and function properly. Unless the accumulated waste is removed, and chronic constipation is corrected, the accumulated waste will slow up the process of healing or, worse, prepare the way for more serious health setbacks. (I would like to digress to add an interesting note: another term for colon irrigation is physic. The origin of the word "physician" is from the Greek word "physika" which means to purge or cleanse.)

Years ago I had an opportunity to talk with Conrad Latto, M.D., who with Dr. Dennis Burkitt, had recently returned from a visit to India. Dr. Burkitt was noted for his research that concluded that a high fiber diet was one of the missing elements in most American and British diets resulting in chronic constipation. The doctors' purpose in going to India was to see if a high fiber diet, consistent with the Indian lifestyle, produced less colon cancer. With the cooperation of the Indian government and the Indian Medical Society, they were able to clinically observe patients regarding how their nutrition affected their colon health. One of the things that Drs. Latto and Burkitt discovered was that most Indian people moved their bowels three times a day. This is a normal process. We eat three times a day; there is good reason why the body should empty its waste from the colon the same number of times. It is Nature's way of keeping the colon clean and healthy. Dr. Latto stated that the colons they observed were in excellent shape, had good muscle tone and good color, thus indicating good blood distribution in this area.

Obviously, these nutritional and lifestyle patterns do not generally pertain to the United States or Great Britain. Three bowel movements a day are more often the exception rather than the rule—and constipation is a widespread condition. When the condition is chronic, or debris has accumulated for years in the colon—as in so many cancer patients—there can be no quick, easy way to repair the problem.

Detoxification Techniques

The process of cleaning the colon and rebuilding muscle tone to restore good peristalsis will require the use of colonics, enemas, roughage and, when necessary, other detoxification procedures. The ordinary enema can be taken at home with the proper equipment. It is a useful way to irrigate the colon and wash out dried fecal contents, even though it cannot reach the areas a high colonic can.

I have found that there is much confusion and controversy surrounding the use of high colonics. High colonics are an effective technique that require the services of a skilled colon therapist. They are done with special equipment, so that water flows in and out of the colon continuously, and is able to reach up into the transverse area instead of just cleaning the descending colon as an enema does. High colonics are particularly useful when the fecal matter has become dry and hard, so that extra effort is needed to eliminate the encrusted waste. A series of high colonics can be an excellent way to improve muscle tone. It would be up to the individual and the professional colon therapist, with the approval of the doctor, to decide whether this is the appropriate procedure for the patient.

There remains a belief in the medical profession that the use of so-called "artificial" procedures such as colonics can paralyze or at least make the colon lazy, so that it will be unable to eliminate wastes on its own. According to this line of reasoning, the sphincter nerve—which is what triggers colon action—is weakened by the colonic. On the contrary, as many natural healers have found through clinic experience, cleansing the hardened waste off the colon wall is the best way to improve muscle tone in order to restore good peristaltic action.

The hostility toward colon cleansing is also based on the argument that irrigations can wash out the healthy intestinal flora which are needed for good elimination. Even if these flora are temporarily washed out, they can easily be replaced by taking naturally fermented foods such as yogurt, clabbered milk or kefir. Another concern of the medical profession is that colon cleansing may create an electrolyte imbalance. In thirty years, I am aware of only one instance where a patient became electrolyte deficient. She caused it by taking colon cleansing for about six consecutive hours. Even this exaggerated use of the colonic, however, did not produce a life-threatening situation. She recovered from the tiredness caused by electrolyte depletion in a matter of hours, by ingesting food containing the missing minerals.

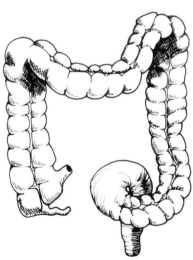

There also are many practitioners of natural healing who oppose colon cleansing, as it violates their concept of natural healing. Under normal circumstances, their view probably would be acceptable but, since the accumulation in the colon is not normal, artificial means of cleansing is the logical way to achieve results.

A Healthy Transverse Colon

Photos courtesy of Victor Earl Irons Company

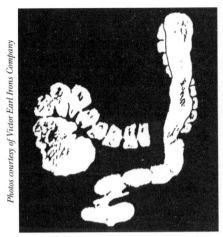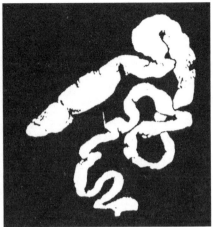

The Distortion of the Unhealthy Colon

I have included above some x-ray photos which show the bulging, twists and other distorted states characteristic of an abnormal colon. The illustration on page 118 shows a healthy colon with normal muscle tone. Often, years of accumulated damage is not easily or quickly repaired, but keeping the colon clean is a first step in that direction. A sound repair program will, of course, also include enough roughage in the diet to help "sweep" the colon clean and reestablish more normal peristaltic movements. These procedures for keeping the colon in good working condition are prerequisites for restoring health and avoiding future complications.

Kidneys

The kidneys are the other major organs of elimination of bodily wastes. In a healthy individual, the kidneys function not only as a filtering system, but also as a means of preserving the body's essential minerals. When, however, the organ becomes exhausted or sluggish in its capability to do its job, the body struggles with excessive biotoxic accumulation. This leads to pollution of the bloodstream, the lymphatics, and other pathologies.

A natural way we can help this biological repair process is to encourage additional elimination of toxic wastes through the kidney by drinking sufficient water. The only water that can be used with a measure of security is distilled water. Contrary to what most people believe, tap water cannot be trusted to be free of chemicals, even though it has been processed to be free of bacteria.

Many individuals who are aware of the toxicity in tap water use well water or spring water instead. But the same complications can exist in well and spring water as in surface water. Some surface water is fed by rain and it is the washout of acid rain which pollutes the reservoir. Because of this almost universal pollution of tap, well water and spring water, we use distilled water as a purer and safer source of liquid. Ample use of distilled water daily to help flush out the body wastes is an excellent way to relieve the kidneys.

From the viewpoint of biological repair, however, the inability of the kidneys to filter the toxic substances from the blood is in itself a reflection of the impairment or breakdown of the waste elimination system as a whole. Kidney function can improve only to the extent that the overall function of the organism is improved by nutrition, detoxification and other biological means.

Skin

This is the largest and often most overlooked organ of elimination. Elimination occurs by way of the pores through perspiration and rashes. Dr. Bernard Jensen, a pioneer in using natural means for restoring health, suggested dry skin-brushing with a natural bristle brush to open up clogged pores. The pores of the skin can get terribly clogged with dirt or dead cells that are constantly being sloughed off and replaced. Soap and water cannot take care of this clogging; the skin brush, made of natural bristles, does an efficient job of opening pores for eliminating toxins. The whole body can be brushed daily with this brush or with a loofah, a type of sponge that can effectively open up the pores. Taking warm baths, with the occasional use of Epsom salts in the water, also encourages skin elimination.

We should avoid antiperspirants as they suppress one of our body's natural areas of elimination. Deodorants may be used as long as they do not contain chemicals. Considering our ever-increasing contamination of air, food and water, it is essential that we keep all avenues of waste elimination open.

The skin is also the largest organ of absorption, therefore, there is a need to protect the skin from the absorption of toxins into the bloodstream. Studies have shown that substances applied on the skin can be measured in the bloodstream within a few minutes. People use all kinds of cosmetics, lotions and creams casually, without realizing that they may contain a number of harmful chemicals that are easily absorbed through the skin and can pollute the entire system.

Lungs

A natural form of elimination that is not always recognized as such is the discharge of mucous, phlegm and other wastes—from a "runny" nose or from the throat. One thing we do not want to do is suppress this elimination with drugs in order to find comfort in the nose and throat.

A healthy alternative is to allow wastes to come out naturally, and to use steam or sweating to speed up the elimination process until the flow of mucus or phlegm subsides on its own. Coughing is still another natural method of expelling waste that should not be suppressed by the use of drugs unless it is causing serious complications. Deliberate coughing is sometimes encouraged to assist the lungs in removing toxicity. The material that is eliminated usually contains dead germs.

We have been operating for too long on a medical system that seeks to ease symptoms rather than deal with the underlying problems. People have been trained to want instant relief instead of tolerating the temporary discomforts that come with symptoms. It is not my purpose here to advise anyone not to use drugs. I believe, however, that if people insist on using drugs, they at least ought to have the privilege of being informed. When knowledgeable, the individual has a free choice and will not make wrong decisions out of ignorance.

Lymphatic System

The lymphatic system is a lesser known pathway of elimination. Vessels of the lymphatic system drain wastes from the the organs. Harmful organisms, when a person's system works properly, will be filtered, attacked, and destroyed. Exercise, jogging, or using a trampoline can stimulate better circulation and increase perspiration. These are excellent ways to cleanse a clogged or backed-up lymphatic system. Or one can use the services of people who are experts in lymphatic massage.

Fasting for Detoxification

I have not as yet discussed a detoxification technique used by some natural-healing practitioners—fasting. Actually, there are two kinds of fasting:

one is the water fast; the other is a liquid fast of diluted vegetable or fruit juices, herbal teas, vegetable broth and distilled water. The two forms of fasting should be carefully differentiated.

The Water Fast

The water fast is a special procedure that is done under the supervision of skilled practitioners and should not be attempted on one's own. The principle behind this technique is that it takes a great deal of energy for the body to go through the full daily digestive process, daily activity—as well as the process of elimination. What the water fast does is lessen considerably the amount of energy that is ordinarily used for a day's activity, making the energy available for healing and elimination of waste (detoxification).

Many practitioners are more than a little uneasy about the water fast for cancer patients. I feel that it was a useful tool at a time when the human system was not absorbing so many toxic pollutants. Today, there can be a risk of complications in this technique—even with professional guidance. Since there are so many toxins in the average body, caused as a result of environmental and nutritional pollution, the water fast can start an accelerated flow of toxins from the cells and tissues. Toxic substances enter the human system in very tiny amounts and get deposited gradually into the tissues and glands. When detoxifying with water alone, the wastes are released into the bloodstream too rapidly, because the body has shifted its energy toward elimination. It is important to be careful that the waste does not move more rapidly than the system of elimination can competently discharge it.

The Juice Fast

The juice fast, on the other hand, is an entirely different procedure. Originated and widely used in European clinics, it was perfected by Are Waerland, Ph.D., as part of a health restoration system that included nutrition and detoxification. During visits to European clinics, I found that there was no hesitation on the part of the doctors to put patients who needed it on a liquid fast containing nutrients—vitamins and minerals. It is a slower detoxification procedure than the water fast, because some of the body's energy goes into digesting the nutrients rather than entirely into the elimination process. This technique is intended to give the body the opportunity to make its biological repairs and to detoxify while it is being nourished with nutrients which are easily digested. As part of this liquid fast, the patient takes enemas morning and night. If the waste products are encouraged to come out of the cells and are collected by the bloodstream, attention has to be given to the actual final elimination process. Liquid fasts can be just as effective as water fasts, and I have not known of a situation where they have been risky for the patient. I observed that many of the patients remained on this liquid fast for a three-week period and some stayed on longer in order to complete their program. A number of the individuals who had never previously heard of fasting were afraid to undertake it at first. Because of their health problems, they hesitated, thinking that perhaps the fast would weaken them further. On the contrary, as a result of the increased elimination of the stored waste, they gained energy. The renewed energy had a general positive effect on the patients' whole mental and physical outlook. After completing the fasts, in fact, many said that they had never felt better in their lives.

Doctors and other practitioners who are experienced in this form of therapy know whether or not the patient requires a fast and if he or she is capable of fasting safely—both of which are important considerations. They are also able to tell, by means of physical symptoms, when the fast has completed its job and should be discontinued. There is a science in bringing people out of a fast properly. Someone who hasn't eaten food for an extended period of time must go back to solids carefully. Indeed, everything is done in a meticulous fashion. An individual should be given enough time to gradually make the transition from fasting to eating; this is the ideal way to derive the most benefit—and to avoid complications.

"Detoxication"

Another more aggressive program for elimination of wastes is Dr. Norman Walker's "detoxication" procedure. This detoxification technique is used when the patient needs to reduce toxicity more aggressively. It utilizes a saline laxative such as Epsom Salts, Glauber's Salts, Pluto Water, or Seidlitz powders. (In general, laxatives should not be used routinely.) The dose should be adequate to stimulate a diarrhea-like movement of the liquid wastes that have been drawn from the lymphatic system.

Because this procedure draws liquid from the glands, fluid replacement is required to avoid dehydration. For this purpose a citrus punch consisting of one half gallon of orange, grapefruit, and lemon juices, plus a half gallon of distilled water, is taken because it enhances the cleansing process. This is done for three consecutive days. The laxatives and the fruit punch fast is followed by another three-day period of combined vegetable juices. After this six-day program, one is considered to have been on a fast, and the fast, therefore, needs to be broken gradually. The first day should consist of raw food only, then a return to the balanced program which includes complex carbohydrates (starches) and proteins.

Many people are under the misunderstanding that an improved dietary regime which includes fruit and vegetable juicing is a form of detoxification. A nutritional program is one thing: it is restorative, it is nourishing; it is also effecting a repair. Detoxification is a separate process. I have tried to show that detoxification can only be said to have occurred in the true sense when waste products are eliminated completely from the body through the colon, kidneys and skin.

Fever: The Body's Own Wisdom

A mechanism that the body uses at times when there is an overload of wastes is to develop a fever. The fact that fever is Nature's own healing process—and not a manifestation of disease—has been determined officially by the National Institute of Allergy and Infectious Diseases (NIAID). Natural practitioners were aware of this more than a century ago. Consequently, they did not attempt to suppress the fever with medications unless the temperature rose to an alarming level (above 104°F). Fever is a natural technique that the body employs to burn up some of the waste products that have accumulated in the system. *Heat also will kill cancer cells.*

Fever is the natural wisdom of the body. When people are feverish, they are usually too tired to go about their regular chores, and so they end up in bed—resting. The energy saved is then converted to healing. Patients don't seem to have an appetite, so there is a natural tendency to fast. And fever creates thirst, so they tend to drink more liquids. As a result, the body is able to rest itself from using energy for the usual day's activity. Thus, it utilizes the rest and extra liquids to flush out some of the burned-up poisons, making them ready for elimination. The body has an innate desire to heal and maintain health, which it will strive to do given the right conditions.

Whole-body hyperthermia is a technique used in a limited number of institutions to produce artificial fever. It is unfortunate that this system is not used as a first choice before employing chemotherapy or radiation, as heat kills cancer cells without doing harm to normal cells (resulting in less damage to the patient). Years ago, *Medical World News* reported on the remarkable results of whole-body hyperthermia in achieving tumor remissions. In the course of the article, it was pointed out that the principle danger of raising the temperature was "that it will prove too effective." When a very large tumor mass is, in effect, dissolved (by the fever), the job of removing the wastes can overwhelm the kidneys. For the most part, the adverse effects of whole-body hyperthermia are relatively mild. For example, a cancer patient with whom I was in touch underwent hyperthermia as part of her repair program. When she returned home, she had breakouts around the mouth area, an indication that the waste that had been stirred up by the heat was not completely eliminated from the body. Nature, in its attempt to finish its work, found another avenue of elimination.

Dr. Pettigrew in Scotland was probably the first physician to employ an original crude method of whole-body hyperthermia (fever therapy). The high temperature he used (110°F) caused the patient's body, according to his report, to break up the cancer cells and other toxins so rapidly that the organs couldn't discard them fast enough through the normal channels of elimination. And so, he writes in his paper, the patients suffered from "kidney crunch." What had happened, in this instance, was that the heat had caused the dead cells to be collected by the bloodstream at too high a concentration for the sluggish eliminatory system to handle. This is an extreme example. It does not ever have to happen. As a matter of fact, Dr. Pettigrew subsequently controlled the cell breakdown to avoid "kidney crunch."

Toxic wastes that have accumulated in the cells can be stored there for a long time before any disease symptoms occur. But if you stir them up too quickly and do not initiate the proper detoxification procedures to remove them from the bloodstream, complications can result. And this, unfortunately, is what can happen when a repair process is in the hands of an amateur.

Biological therapies can stimulate the cells and tissues to release the toxins they have absorbed and have been storing for a long time. To clear up one of the main confusions that may arise, I need to point out that detoxification does not consist merely of the process of bringing toxins from the cellular or glandular level into the bloodstream. The fact that this has been accomplished does not necessarily mean that the toxic wastes are eliminated automatically through the anus. It usually needs help to accomplish the final elimination.

People should not think that merely changing their diet means they are detoxifying. It is true that by doing this they are encouraging the cells to discard stored-up waste products. And any number of biological repairs which I have mentioned previously—spinal manipulation, adjusting the temporomandibular joint, massage, even simple exercising—can start that action. When we say detoxification, we really and truly mean final elimination of wastes from the body via the colon. Unless these toxins are cleared out of the body by way of the eliminatory passageways, they may recirculate back to the bloodstream.

There is a profound difference between starting the wastes moving from the cells into the bloodstream—and actually getting rid of them by way of the colon, primarily, or through the skin by sweating or by kidney elimination. This difference must be understood when one initiates a biorepair. As all skilled practitioners know from experience, it is wise to place the patient on a detoxification regimen even before they undertake a biological therapy. Otherwise, if the cells are stimulated to give up the wastes they have been storing—and the body doesn't eliminate them—they can cause the bloodstream to be polluted.

I hope that it is evident that the proper elimination of accumulated wastes is indispensable for any program that seeks to repair the biological impairments and breakdowns involved in cancer and other degenerative diseases. A body that has been repeatedly subjected to toxic products beyond its capacity to eliminate them will need considerable help to detoxify safely and efficiently. When the detoxification techniques described in this chapter are combined with other biological therapies, the benefits are greatly enhanced.

7. Some Psychological Considerations

It isn't the burdens of today that drive men mad.
It is the regrets over yesterday and the fear of tomorrow.
Regret and fear are twin thieves who rob us of today.
—ROBERT J. HASTINGS

f it is true that cancer is caused by biological and psychological problems affecting the whole body, it is equally true that recovery is the process of repairing the body in its entirety. I hope I've already made it clear that the human system is so interrelated in its workings that a physical dysfunction in one area can have a negative effect on other areas. Conversely, an improvement in one function can help the whole system get better. The interrelationship pertains, of course, to the psychological as well as physical aspects of a patient's life.

When dealing with degenerative diseases such as cancer, we have to realize that for the majority of patients, all factors, physical and psychological, must be considered relative if the repair program is to restore the patient's health. Some practitioners who advocate single-substance therapy have on occasion helped a patient, but improvement may not be sustained as the root cause was not corrected. There probably isn't an alternative system which doesn't show some improvement for someone, although it may be limited. Because of this initial improvement, people assume they have the universal therapy that is right for everyone.

A successful cancer therapy is one that takes into account the whole body and mind; has a clinically proven pattern of repair; uses non-toxic, non-invasive, diagnostic methods to find out where the biological breakdown is and what is causing it; and then addresses the problems with an integrated repair program of biological therapy. In addition, a sound therapy has to demonstrate success for a large group of people with a variety of cancer types over a period of at least ten years before it should be considered viable. In this type of biological approach, the practitioner sees to it that the patient's system is nourished at the cellular level and emotional factors are addressed. Emphasis must also be put on waste elimination to get the cells to give up their storage of poor quality materials and toxins, and restoration of normal biological function. All possible areas requiring attention should be given consideration, whether it is nutritional, structural, glandular or emotional.

Far too often we run across the narrow-minded therapeutic approach which zeroes in on one single factor to the exclusion of others. For example, there are those in the psychological field who tend to attribute cancer to emotional distress alone, and assume that correcting this problem will be the total solution. This concept is just as one-dimensional as the nutritionist who thinks that a better diet is going to be the sole panacea, or the practitioner who does spinal manipulation in the belief that once he accomplishes the alignment, the patient will surely recover. One may indeed come across an individual who gets well as a result of this single-minded therapy, but only because in that one very rare instance the treatment affected the sole cause of the problem. But how is this approach going to help the vast numbers of cancer patients who almost invariably have gotten cancer from a number of other causes, psychological as well as physical?

I have never said that the biological approach to repair—which tries to take into account all of the factors we have mentioned—will save every patient's life. But I do know from experience that biological therapies have proven successful for many people and have provided immeasurable improvement in many instances where other approaches have failed. There are times, unfortunately, when the individual's breakdown is too extreme to be reversed by means of any therapy or the psychological need for the illness has been left uncorrected. Yet one should always remember that the body has enormous healing capability.

In previous chapters I have dealt in-depth with the two most important aspects of biological therapy—nutrition and detoxification. In the following pages, I will discuss psychological factors that should be considered if the patient is to derive the greatest possible benefit from his or her repair program.

THE PSYCHOLOGICAL DIMENSION

There is no doubt that the patient's psychological attitude plays a profound role in the recovery program. It can be a factor that interferes with, or hastens the process of restoring health. Studies have shown, for example, that many individuals who develop cancer often have a lifelong emotional pattern that includes a sense of hopelessness and helplessness, lack of self-esteem, depression, anxiety, repressed anger, or a need for self punishment. These negative emotions that underlie a patient's personality can undermine the course of the best repair regimen, just as a positive system of emotions can help the patient maintain a relaxed body that allows it to function optimally.

Although I am not trained in psychology, I constantly see and therefore cannot ignore the more subtle ways in which a patient's destructive psychological pattern can sabotage and undermine his or her own health. There is, for instance, the type of individual who is always verbalizing that he is going to get well, but is constantly doing things to undermine a recovery. Or else, they will secretly do things they know perfectly well are not acceptable on a biological repair regime and then tell the practitioner afterward about the abuse. I am thinking of one individual in particular who subjected herself to a brain scan, with all of the negative aspects of unnecessary radiation, even though there was no indication that the scan was required. I asked her why she had done this, knowing that it would be better to avoid unnecessary radiation. Her answer was, "Well, I suppose I was just curious." It is as if this was her deliberate intention—to make the move first and then to call after she had violated the biological concept of avoiding unnecessary radiation.

I can illustrate this with another example, this one of a patient with colon cancer whose condition had improved considerably in the course of a biological therapy to the extent that her bleeding had stopped completely. This woman called FACT after a six-month silence to inform us that she was unable to move her bowels at all, and that she was terrified because the bleeding had resumed.

When I asked why she hadn't been in touch with her doctor all along, and had waited until this problem could no longer be ignored, she answered that she had discontinued the nutrition/detoxification program when the bleeding had stopped. In the course of the conversation, she also revealed that she had gone through extensive x-rays of the mouth, even though only one tooth was involved and required only one or two x-rays at the most. Yet she had allowed this to be done, knowing that the last thing she needed was to have her whole mouth unnecessarily radiated. I pointed out to this woman that it took at least a two-year process to effect a biological repair and that she had stopped the process long before her impaired system had been corrected. Because of this, her body continued to produce cancer cells and the symptoms that went along with it. "Don't you realize," I asked her, "that you are the one who is in total charge of what you are doing, and how casual you have been about a dangerous disease that needs to be taken with the utmost seriousness?" "Well," was her answer, "I guess I have always taken a 'what will be will be' attitude toward life, and this is no exception."

This patient is by no means unusual. There are others too who begin a metabolic program, stop after a period of some success, and lose touch with FACT and their practitioner until some alarming problem resurfaces. Whatever their psychological motivation, there is not much that can be done with individuals who proceed down their own destructive road until it is too late to reverse the damage unless they include psychological counseling as part of the regimen. It is not within my ability—nor is it my role— to analyze where this attitude comes from. Undoubtedly, it is a deeply rooted pattern of behavior that is different in each individual.

Whatever their original psychological background might be, some patients have a tremendous drive to get well and some do not. I know people who have been able to overcome a very serious breakdown while others, however, who were not nearly as ill, continued to decline because they were not motivated toward survival. There comes to mind a patient who maintained a tumor for more than twenty-three years, even though her practitioner had given her the kind of program that would enhance her chances of complete tumor reduction. Of course, the tumor wouldn't dissolve, since she didn't consistently follow a metabolic regimen although she was knowledgeable enough to do so. Being a cancer patient brought her a great deal of sympathy from the people around her, and such a lifelong craving for attention seemed to be controlling her actions. She could have benefited from expert psychological counseling; yet, in her case, I did not feel she would die of cancer without counseling as indeed she did not. I believe her motivation was simply sympathy. (She died twenty-three years after the initial diagnosis at the age of 83, not of cancer but of heart failure.)

People don't realize that negative motivation can be just as powerful a factor as positive motivation. An individual's subconscious goal may be to die, because of chronic depression, lack of goals or values, or being fed up to the point where life no longer seems worth living. Another person may just want to get constant love from the family, or punish a loved one for a real or imagined hurt. Whatever their psychological reason, what better way to achieve their goal than to sabotage their own recovery? To gain control over one's destructive motives, professional psychological guidance would be a positive direction to squelch the demon. Situations such as I have described do exist. And if they do, the only way to reverse a self-destructive drive is by finding a new direction—and that is where counseling can usually be of great help.

On the other hand, the fact is that many positive individuals possess a will to survive that carries them successfully through all stages of the biological repair process. Appendix I relates the experiences of a number of cancer patients whose determination—perhaps "life force" is a better term—helped them overcome the most extraordinary obstacles in their pathway to recovery. I often give the illustration of a man I knew who was afflicted with cancer of the spine. It had reached the stage where his spine could no longer support his body, so that he was reduced to lying on his back, with little or no hope of reversing his condition. Yet, in this supine state, he did what most individuals would not have had the courage to do. On his own, he signed himself out of the hospital, went home and with the help of a knowledgeable friend began to read up on the biological repair process. The book he used was *How to Always Be Well* by William Howard Hay, M.D. This anecdote provides an inkling of an individual's strong will to get well. Gradually, he started to regain his health by applying some of these biological ideas to his own condition. He went on a metabolic and waste elimination program and—with the physical assistance of his wife and the help of a physician experienced in natural healing—slowly began to accomplish the repair. From being flat on his back, he struggled into a position where he was able to sit up with a brace; then he used a wheelchair; next he used crutches; then a walker until he could manage to get around quite nicely, at first with a cane and then on his own. He was self-motivated—and through his own efforts fought hard to get himself back into a state of health. He died at the age of 84 of natural causes, twenty-seven years from the time of the original diagnosis.

It must be realized, too, that in addition to the weight of psychological problems of the past, the cancer patient is suddenly confronted with a whole new emotional dynamic of fear, pain and doubts about his or her ability to recover. The reluctance of some cancer patients to truly accept the reality of their situation as a life-or-death-struggle for survival, in which there will be uncomfortable healing flare-ups as well as periods of well-being, is entirely understandable. It is never easy to change one's life pattern and doubly difficult when one is burdened by the debilitating physical and emotional weight of cancer.

Practitioners realize from long experience that educating the patient to recognize and overcome psychological resistance is an integral part of the repair program. They take into consideration the situational factors that make for resistance, and try to set up a realistic program that does not confront the patient with too many sudden demands that might prove counterproductive. As the patient gains confidence in one area, and begins to feel better, he or she can then undertake more responsibility for fulfilling the various aspects of the overall regime. The patients ultimately learn that, in the final analysis, the job of getting well is in their hands.

Sometimes it is quite evident that the individual could benefit from psychological guidance. I do not feel, however, that patients who are emotionally troubled should undertake deep psychotherapy during the repair process. Probing for the lifelong factors that underlie emotional problems is not appropriate at a time when the patient is trying to affect a biological repair, because the turmoil stirred up by this form of treatment may be too much for the individual to handle with all the other responsibilities. They need behavioral therapy more than any other type until the repair is effected. This can be of great value in helping them repattern their destructive lifestyle and see how their current actions undercut the therapy. After they regain their health sufficiently, they may wish to probe into the basic reasons why they are functioning psychologically as they do.

I strongly suggest that the individual who needs emotional help get counseling from a person who is also familiar with the concepts of biorepair; some counselors feel that a patient needs to face the reality of cancer as a death sentence. When one is on a biorepair program, facing death is not the appropriate direction.

STRESS MANAGEMENT

I have noted that when a condition of extreme stress is allowed to continue unabated, it can exhaust the individual's system and distort normal body functions. The endocrine secretions that the body emits become too skewed under stress to keep the body chemistry in balance. The nervous system is overstimulated; heart rate and blood pressure may be increased or depressed; digestion and elimination are off balance, therefore, foods are not metabolized properly, thus making the micronutrients unavailable for cell production. At some point, an individual's chronic stress can cause any number of diseases and unless corrected may make it virtually impossible for the biorepair to take place.

Biofeedback

Very often it has been useful for patients to use biofeedback or meditation to reduce stress, as it helps deflect the tension from having a negative impact on body function. Once the stress is sufficiently controlled, it allows a more harmonious functioning of the body, so that the repair process can resume. These techniques do not deal in depth with the patient's underlying psychological problems. That is the function of a psychotherapist. What biofeedback and meditation can do, however, is enable the patient to decrease the effect of stress on body function. It is useful as a palliative procedure which is needed to allow the body to function efficiently until more in-depth procedures are undertaken.

There are biofeedback centers where people can be taught control procedures with mechanical equipment to measure the change in their automatic responses. Through their experience with patients, biofeedback professionals have found that the principal causes of stress are: death of a loved one; serious illness; divorce or the breakup of an important relationship; despair or deep fear about children; loss of job or home; and relocation or economic problems. You cannot assume, however, that all stress is emotionally induced. There are tensions that can be created because the body is in a toxic state which plays havoc with nerves. If the cause is toxicity, no matter how much psychotherapy or biofeedback is done, only partial relief may be attained. Until the toxicity is eliminated from the patient's system, the stress itself will not be alleviated. The mind and the body are interlinked; the mind can wreak havoc on the body and, conversely, the body can wreak havoc on the mind.

Physical/Emotional Link

There is a dramatic example which underlines the influence of the physical on the emotional. It concerns schizophrenia, which is not considered curable through psychological counseling. I came across an article about a schizophrenia patient who needed kidney dialysis. After undergoing treatment, the young man was not only relieved of toxicity in the bloodstream due to kidney failure, but his schizophrenic symptoms disappeared! It was quite a revelation! It was obvious that the man's mind had been affected by his toxic bloodstream. Thus, in this case, stress management was a detoxification procedure.

Some time after reading about this, I introduced two oncologists, Dr. Donald Cole and Dr. John Pung, to a piece of equipment called a Hemadetoxifier, manufactured by Becton Dickinson, a pharmaceutical supply company. The Hemadetoxifier is designed to enable oncologists to detoxify the bloodstream if a cancer patient receives a dangerous overdose of chemotherapy. Becton Dickinson supplied the equipment without cost. Their profit was derived from the sale of the charcoal-filled canisters which become polluted with the toxic waste and have to be discarded after each use.

Through an organization of parents of schizophrenics, I learned of a young man who was making life very difficult for his family. He was under the care of a psychiatrist who prescribed Thorazine but he was still hard to control. I suggested detoxification and told them about the experience the schizophrenic had with dialysis. I also suggested that they could try detoxification with Drs. Cole and Pung. They agreed.

The young man had been irrational and on Thorazine, a behavior-controlling drug, for a long time. He was uncooperative and had to be given a mild sedative just to calm him so he would lie down long enough to be treated. After his bloodstream was cleansed, he sat up smiling and thanked everyone, including his psychiatrist who attended in order to see the results. The detoxification was a success. The chap's behavior became rational. This one detoxification allowed him to function normally, without drugs, for nearly eighteen months. Toward the end of this period the irrational behavior pattern gradually recurred. (No doubt during this period he returned to his habitual lifestyle and his bloodstream became toxic again.) Even this one example points up the fact that the detoxification process may be valuable in treating other problems related to toxicity as well as cancer. What we cannot ignore is the effect of physical factors on the psychological condition.

Meditational Techniques

Meditation can help to alleviate the effects of stress on the body. I am sympathetic with this technique, not so much as a spiritual philosophy, but as a means of getting the body to relax, so that the tensions of the day do not play havoc with the physical being and upset the metabolic process. There are a number of good books on the subject and centers in large cities that teach simple meditational procedures. Meditation in its various forms provides a calming atmosphere, free of external distractions, in which the individual experiences a decrease in metabolic, brain wave and endocrine activity. Research studies show that during the meditational state—when the individual's attention is restricted to limited stimuli—there is a reduction in oxygen consumption, respiratory rate, heart rate and blood pressure. This pattern of lowered physiological activity has been called the "relaxation response."

PEACE OF MIND

There is also another aspect of living that ought to be recognized as a biological need—and that is what has most often been called "peace of mind." Different people achieve this state of being and feeling in different ways—through hobbies or holidays, meditating or reading, listening to music or Nature walks. Whatever satisfies the individual, bringing him or her in closer touch with the self, can be a means of finding peace of mind.

And this, of course, brings up the related state of experiencing joy of living. An individual who is very ill is not going to make the necessary effort to get well unless there is a feeling that life has value, that it has beauty, that it has things to offer beyond routine everyday experiences. The value that individuals place upon their lives, their interest in people and things outside themselves, will have a profound bearing on their will to survive. If, for instance, there is a death in the family, some patients will react to the loss with a feeling of being utterly lonesome and deprived, so that their health begins to slide downhill. Others in the same tragic circumstances can be alone without being lonesome, finding all sorts of worthwhile activities to fill their lives.

Even the most painful of situations need not rob an individual of the feeling that life is still worth living. On the other hand, if the cancer patient says, "What is the point of life, why should I fight to restore my health?"— chances are they will not survive. This point of view is well illustrated in the book, *Your Body Believes Every Word You Say* by Barbara Levine.

I am reminded, as I write this, of an elderly cancer patient who entered an old age home. She could have taken the easy way out—given in to a sense of despair, not because she was afraid that she would not get well, but because it was a situation in which many people think that life is useless. This woman, however, made the best of her circumstances, felt satisfaction in her new friends, activities and entertainment, and the people who were there to encourage and serve her. Somehow she had found within herself a life force that kept her alive long after many others would have succumbed.

How does one motivate patients who do not find a sense of purpose within themselves to continue the fight for the preservation of life? I wish I could say that one can readily provide such individuals with a motivation—a cause, a moral or spiritual direction. People can be helped up to a point—sometimes through a counselor—but they also need to have some inner sense of courage or curiosity and zest for life. The opportunity exists for all of us to find and involve ourselves in some form of meaningful activity. I have known cancer patients who, even in the most difficult of circumstances, have somehow made the time and found the energy to get involved with others, devote themselves to social or political work, do art, music or crafts. For the most part, they are involved in these activities to fulfill themselves, not because someone has suggested that they find an outside interest.

But it is not easy to discern during the repair process whether or not a patient is motivated to succeed. The fact that some individuals do recover and fulfill their life expectancy is a tribute to their resourcefulness in carrying out the healing program and—equally as important—their indomitable will to survive.

PATIENT-FAMILY RELATIONSHIPS

From my observations—and the experiences of practitioners—a program does not seem to work out competently when a member of the family attempts to impose it on the patient and make decisions for them. Patients need to be self-motivated and make their own decisions, even though they seem to be wrong to others. The feeling of being in control is essential for the patients' well-being in carrying out a biological repair program. We cannot know, of course, what the psychological ramifications of a family relationship may be. On the surface it may appear to be a positive and cooperative relationship; what goes on between them on a deeper level may be another matter entirely. However, one thing has to be clearly understood: the health restoration situation is one in which the cancer patient must be an active participant and assume much of the responsibility for his or her actions. There must be no way for the patient to lay the blame for anything that occurs on anyone else. Nor should the patient be given the opportunity to use his or her illness as a means of taking revenge for some real or imaginary hurt by a family member.

I am reminded of a case where the husband, a thoughtful and caring human being, had taken on complete responsibility for his wife's health. He was the one who called FACT, reported on her progress in order to find out the appropriate therapy, or what referral she ought to have. I repeatedly told him that he was playing a harmful role, and that this was not an appropriate position for him. I advised him to encourage his wife to decide what she wanted to do and to what degree she would adhere to the repair procedure. The control needed to be in his wife's hands, with her making all the calls to her practitioner. If she was capable of speaking—and of course she was—she was the one who should be in charge of her recovery. Otherwise, if the treatment seems to be ineffective, she can always blame her husband: "You were the one who told me to do this" or, "You gave me the wrong information" or, "It's your fault that I'm not getting well."

It is even conceivable that her motivation—hidden even to herself—was to make certain that the repair program failed, or to state it differently, he failed. Perhaps there was always resentment against his being successful or dominant, and there was a drive in her to make him fail in this instance. In spite of his devotion and diligent care and the fact that physiologically she was a good candidate for recovery, she died.

One can never know the tangled and complex emotional forces that exist between two close individuals—only that they can exist and make for all kinds of complications. Whatever the underlying reasons may be, I have rarely known a successful instance where one member of a family completely took over the choices of another. The only thing a husband, wife, child or loved one can do is to serve, but not dominate, the cancer patient. It may be difficult for the patient or the family to accept this reality, but unless they do, the healing process can be impeded or even made impossible.

The vitality of the human body is not only dependent upon physical factors such as nutrition and waste elimination, but also emotional well-ness. The power of the mind to either encourage or hinder healing should not be ignored. Self-destructive habits and self-defeating thoughts can prevent recovery; optimism and hope are necessary for repair. Cancer patients should not struggle with psychological issues but resolve them with an appropriate therapist or counselor. I hope that I have emphasized the need to treat the mind, as well as the body, when repairing a biological breakdown.

8. Some Physical Considerations

Health is so necessary to all the duties as well as the pleasures of life, that the crime of squandering it is equal to the folly.
—Dr. Samuel Johnson

Since there was an overview of physical considerations in a previous chapter and knowing that I will be repeating myself in some instances, I want to present a more in-depth understanding of what can break down how repairs can be made and the importance of making those repairs. Some areas that are given too little consideration by patients can have a serious negative impact on a repair program if neglected.

SPINAL ALIGNMENT

Practitioners who are involved with biological therapies are aware that a misaligned spinal column can impede a biorepair. As previously stated, the various organs are signaled into activity by means of the nerve network and the autonomic nerve system, which works automatically and spontaneously. The nerve endings relating to their associated organs are situated between the spinal vertebrae. If an individual has poor posture or develops a curvature or other abnormal condition of the spine, it may impinge on instructions from the brain to the related organ. As a consequence, the bowel, circulation, lungs, endocrine secretions, etc. will not function efficiently.

It is always wise for a repair program to incorporate corrective techniques for spinal alignment, whether by an osteopathic physician or a chiropractor. There is a difference between the two disciplines. Both are concerned with the same problems in general, but their techniques and training differ. The osteopath undergoes the rigorous training required for a medical degree plus the added discipline of manipulation, whereas, the chiropractor is trained primarily in a system of manipulation that varies from that of an osteopath.

Osteopathic or chiropractic adjustments usually include muscle relaxation, glandular stimulation and drainage, breathing to bring oxygen to the apices to provide sufficient oxygen for the bloodstream, nerve relaxation and, in some instances, cranial adjustments.

TEMPOROMANDIBULAR JOINT (TMJ)

The temporomandibular joint is located just in front of the ear, facilitating the articulation of the lower jaw. It is not sufficiently understood that the displacement of this joint can create impairments seemingly unrelated to a dental malocclusion. More doctors are beginning to practice wholistic medicine; therefore, more attention to all of the physical areas that impinge on normal function (including the TMJ) that might be hampering the harmonious functioning of the body is taken into consideration. Although a great deal of research and writing has been done about TMJ problems, especially by William B. May, D.D.S., only a limited group in the medical profession recognize the role of the displaced mandible in causing low back pains, headaches, tinnitus, and a wide range of other ailments. It cuts off circulation to the eyes which can result in macular degeneration.

It is not widely realized that a misaligned TMJ can create enormous problems along the spinal column which in turn blocks signals to the related organs, upsets the nerve system, and impairs metabolism and other vital body functions. Because the displacement causes weakening of the signals to the organs of metabolism, it impairs the breakdown of food into microcomponents essential for healthy cell production.

A dentist, cranial osteopath or cranial chiropractor can decide whether the misalignment exists and try to manipulate the joint back into its proper rotating position. Through feedback from patients who have undergone this corrective procedure, it seems to be preferable to have a dentist carefully calibrate the malocclusion and place a corrective, removable plastic splint in place to maintain the proper occlusion. This plastic splint can be taken out whenever one talks or eats, and is worn at other times during the day or night. By creating proper occlusion, the splint realigns the jaw joint, and the muscles then relax so that the circulatory and nerve blockages are relieved.

Wearing the splint for a period of time usually makes it possible for the impeded signals to connect to the related organs, and the symptoms associated with the displaced TMJ will disappear. And once the joint problem is repaired, the spine can continue to hold its proper position after the spinal misalignment has been corrected. It is hard for most people to comprehend how a joint in the jaw can affect the spinal column—and, indeed, the whole biological process—but you can see this network of nerve connections if you study the chart on pages 142–143.

Repairing the TMJ should be considered as essential as nutrition, waste elimination, stress control and so forth. I recently referred a man, who had been unable to correct a hearing difficulty for years, to a dentist who specialized in TMJ work. It turned out that his deafness was due to the misaligned temporomandibular joint. Soon after the adjustment had been completed, he went outside his home to set out his trash. A neighbor who was doing the same thing asked him a question and as he answered, he realized to his astonishment that he was able to hear without his hearing aid. I have learned too, that some cancer patients cannot be helped substantially, even when they are on a sound repair program, until this joint is adjusted.

PHYSICAL FITNESS

A good exercise regime that is right for the individual is as important to his or her body as any other need. Without sufficient physical activity, our muscles would atrophy, our oxygen supply would be deficient, and the body's heart and lung system would suffer. Exercise is beneficial towards helping improve bad posture, stimulating glandular flow and keeping the waste elimination process active.

Physical activity does not have to be strenuous to be effective. We need only exercise to the point of limbering our muscles, not to the point of exhaustion. The right exercise technique provides relaxation and builds energy. Exhausting or strenuous exercise has a negative effect. It diverts vitality from other normal body processes such as digestion, elimination of waste, absorption and healing. All one has to do is find a suitable exercise regime that will help keep the muscles supple. Muscles pertain to not only the obvious external musculature, but the internal musculature as well—the colon is made up of muscles, as are the kidneys, the bladder, the heart,

Chart of the

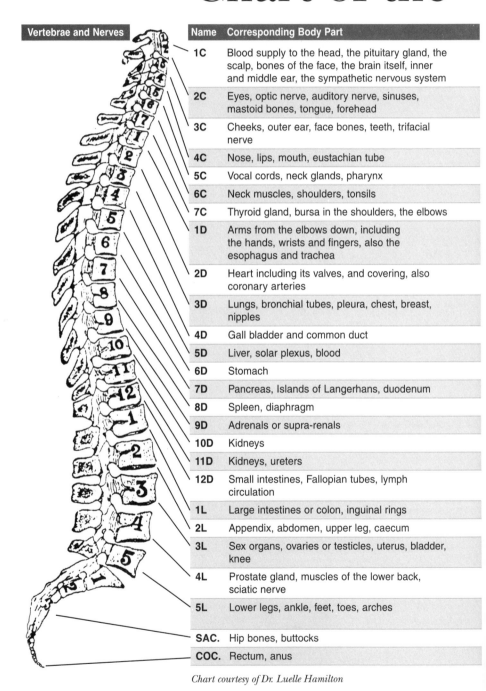

Name	Corresponding Body Part
1C	Blood supply to the head, the pituitary gland, the scalp, bones of the face, the brain itself, inner and middle ear, the sympathetic nervous system
2C	Eyes, optic nerve, auditory nerve, sinuses, mastoid bones, tongue, forehead
3C	Cheeks, outer ear, face bones, teeth, trifacial nerve
4C	Nose, lips, mouth, eustachian tube
5C	Vocal cords, neck glands, pharynx
6C	Neck muscles, shoulders, tonsils
7C	Thyroid gland, bursa in the shoulders, the elbows
1D	Arms from the elbows down, including the hands, wrists and fingers, also the esophagus and trachea
2D	Heart including its valves, and covering, also coronary arteries
3D	Lungs, bronchial tubes, pleura, chest, breast, nipples
4D	Gall bladder and common duct
5D	Liver, solar plexus, blood
6D	Stomach
7D	Pancreas, Islands of Langerhans, duodenum
8D	Spleen, diaphragm
9D	Adrenals or supra-renals
10D	Kidneys
11D	Kidneys, ureters
12D	Small intestines, Fallopian tubes, lymph circulation
1L	Large intestines or colon, inguinal rings
2L	Appendix, abdomen, upper leg, caecum
3L	Sex organs, ovaries or testicles, uterus, bladder, knee
4L	Prostate gland, muscles of the lower back, sciatic nerve
5L	Lower legs, ankle, feet, toes, arches
SAC.	Hip bones, buttocks
COC.	Rectum, anus

Vertebrae and Nerves

Chart courtesy of Dr. Luelle Hamilton

Nerve System

Heaches, nervousnes, insomnia, head colds, high blood pressure, migraine headaches, mental conditions, nervous breakdown, amnesia, epilepsy, infantile paralysis, sleeping sickness, chronic tiredness, dizziness or vertigo, St. Vitus dance

Sinus trouble, allergies, crossed eyes, deafness, erysipelas, eye troubles, earache, fainting spells, certain cases of blindness

Neuralgia, neuritis, acne or pimples, eczema

Hay fever, rose fever, etc, catarrh, hard of hearing, adenoids

Laryngitis, hoarseness, throat conditions like a sore throat, quinsy, etc

Stiff neck, pain in upper arm, tonsilitis, whooping cough, croup

Bursitis, colds, thyroid conditions, goiter

Asthma, cough, difficult breathing, shortness of breath, pain in lower arms and hands

Functional heart conditions and certain chest pains

Bronchitis, pleurisy, pneumonia, congestion, influenza, grippe

Gall bladder conditions, jaundice, shingles

Liver conditions, fevers, low blood pressure, anemia, poor circulation, arthritis

Stomach troubles including nervous stomach, indigestion, heart burn, dyspepsia, etc.

Diabetes, ulcers, gastritis

Leukemia, hiccoughs

Allergies, hives

Kidney troubles, hardening of the arteries, chronic tiredness, nephritis, pyelitis

Skin conditions like acne, or pimples, eczema, boils, etc., auto-intoxication

Rheumatism, gas pains, certain types of sterility

Constipation, colitis, dysentery, diarrhea, ruptures of hernias

Appendicitis, cramps, difficult breathing, acidosis, varicose veins

Bladder troubles, menstrual troubles like painful or irregular periods, miscarriages, bed wetting, impotency, change of life symptoms, many knee pains

Sciatica, lumbago, difficult, painful or too frequent urination, backaches

Poor circulation in the legs, swollen ankles, weak ankles and arches, cold feet, weakness in the legs, leg cramps

Sacro-illiac condition, spinal curvatures

Hemmoroids or piles, pruritus or itching, pain at end of spine on sitting

*Very few of the conditions listed wholly within the control of any one special nerve. Only the more common conditions and diseases are listed.

the lungs. All these organs have to be kept toned if they are to perform their various functions as effectively as they should.

If one's normal life activities are sufficient to keep the muscles in good shape, that is fine; no additional exercises may be needed. That is, however, a rare situation in our society. For the most part, people have sedentary jobs. If you find yourself in this situation, there are a wide range of conditioning activities to which you can devote some time on a regular basis. It need not be long hours or exhausting.

Aerobics, walking or swimming and body-tensing exercises, or isometrics, fit into categories of good exercises for patients, since they are not too overtaxing, yet keep the muscles in good shape. (An aerobic exercise is one that involves the whole body and increases heart rate and oxygen consumption over a sustained period of time.) Though most people don't realize it, walking is probably the easiest, most convenient, and efficient exercise to help people get in shape and stay in good condition. Swimming, too, engages all of the muscles and keeps the body buoyant and relaxed. These gentle exercises help condition the muscles, strengthen the heart and lungs, increase stamina, improve food absorption and utilization, and stimulate better elimination. As an added benefit, the aftermath of exercise is to reduce tension and anxiety, and make for more restful sleep.

Simple yoga postures and exercises are truly excellent ways to stretch and loosen up the muscles and make them more elastic. Their aim, according to those who espouse the yoga philosophy, is also to normalize the physiological and spiritual functions of the human organism as a whole. There are books which provide easy-to-follow yoga programs for home practice, and centers where inexpensive instruction is available.

Doing slant board exercises is a method of changing the normal pull of gravity by placing your body at an angle in which the head is below the feet. This is a good way to get better circulation throughout the entire body and especially into the head, reaching areas that are not ordinarily open. There are instructions for the beginner; none of these exercises need to be overdone to be beneficial.

Another technique which patients have found to be useful is to use mini-trampolines (sometimes called rebounders). They replace the need to jog on hard cement surfaces, a jolting experience for the body. These small trampolines consist of tough plastic surfaces held to a low steel frame with springs. The individual bounces on this resilient surface, providing stimulation to the bottom of the feet. These relaxed bouncing movements engage all the muscles of the body without jarring or strain. This is a good, gentle form of physical activity that stimulates the lymphatics, expands the lungs and keeps the muscles limber. It is especially good for patients who need exercise but do not have the energy or time for outdoor activities.

There are a number of different mini-trampolines on the market; I do not recommend one over another. They are all competent enough. Unfortunately, because of the over commercialization of the whole health field, and the number of people who are desperately searching for panaceas, exaggerated claims are made for all kinds of products, which we feel are not warranted.

The question sometimes arises as to whether cancer patients, who may not be too well physically, should exercise. Yes. There are bedridden people who have been encouraged to exercise to keep their muscles from getting too flabby. They can, for example, press their feet against the mattress, or raise their hands above their head and over to the sides. There are body-tensing exercises (isometrics) which are quite helpful in toning the muscles. It is wise to include exercise in all repair programs. In addition to its effect on improving the physical condition, exercise is psychologically important as well, giving the patient the rewarding sense of being in touch with his or her own body and releasing endorphins.

BREATHING

Many people are unaware that they have gotten into the bad habit of shallow breathing. People under great stress, for example, can actually neglect to breathe in the normal fashion, which involves completely expanding the lung capacity. An individual can actually make deep breathing a conscious activity until the body does it automatically.

It is for good reason that breath has been called the essence of life. Oxygen is a vital factor in maintaining the metabolic activities of every cell, tissue and organ system. Where there is an inadequate supply of this nutrient, the proper molecular exchange between the nutritive substances in the food and the cells cannot take place. The result can be a serious interference with the processes of oxygenation, waste exchange, cell renewal, repair and survival. Dr. Otto Warburg is well known for his research which concluded that cancer cells cannot survive in an oxygenated environment; therefore, it can be of tremendous benefit to the body's healing effort to deliberately and conscientiously include breathing exercises in a biorepair program.

LIGHT AND HEALTH

The importance light plays in human health is increasingly being recognized. Sunlight is a factor that, along with food, water, air and rest, makes possible the life support system on earth. Just as plants need light for photosynthesis, human beings require a certain amount of natural light to carry out life processes normally.

Exposure to sunlight stimulates the development of vitamin D, which is stored in the body and is automatically available to be utilized for a number of vital functions. Recent studies have found that light actually is helpful in preventing and treating some diseases, is essential to the endocrine system's activity, encourages growth, lessens stress and improves behavior patterns. In addition, the effect of sunlight is that of a natural psychological tranquilizer, which can reduce tension and anxiety.

There is sometimes a mistaken resistance to sun exposure by cancer patients because of the knowledge that sunlight can be harmful to the skin. It may indeed be, if the individual is exposed to the rays of the sun for too long a period of time. Like everything else, sunlight should be taken in moderate amounts. Typically, when people feel that the sun is a great healer, they tend to saturate their bodies with an excessive amount. Instead of overdoing or entirely neglecting sunlight, there is a sensible time of exposure which Nature intended and that our bodies will appreciate. Since this area of moderation is so wide and gives you so much latitude, I cannot understand why so many people manage to find the dangerous extremes—too much or too little.

Though sunlight is the finest source of light, there are alternate ways to get the full spectrum light that we need for our health. A full spectrum fluorescent bulb of special design which duplicates natural light is available. This is a very useful device for people who must spend much of their day under artificial light, in the form of incandescent or ordinary fluorescent bulbs. The absence of full spectrum light—or malillumination as it has been termed—can produce malaise, just as any interference with normal life processes can. Dr. John Ott, a pioneer in light research for fifty years, and author of *Health and Light*, has warned about the harmful effects of excessive artificial light. It is his belief, validated by extensive research using time-lapse photography that shows growth or impaired growth, that sunlight is one of the important survival factors in human life.

When a cancer patient holds a job where the lights are artificial, they should make every effort to have access to a full spectrum source, no matter how this is accomplished. Patients who are bedridden or must spend a great deal of time indoors should also have access to full spectrum light, during the winter as well as the summer months. The use of such a light source is a good solution to the problem of obtaining sufficient quality light when there is limited availability of natural sunlight.

REST

Adequate sleep and rest would seem to be an obvious aspect of health that needs no discussion. Yet, the fact is that many people who deal quite conscientiously with their body's natural requirements, violate—really violate—the biological rule of rest. Some patients, for example, who are still on a regular work schedule will stay up late into the night, then use an alarm clock to wake them up early in the morning. In doing this, they are abruptly disturbing their sleep cycle before it is complete. Or else, they interrupt their sleep in order to work on a project, instead of first getting sufficient sleep and then tackling the project when they are ready for it.

What these individuals don't seem to understand is that healing takes place during rest, and that each human system has its own unique requirements for the amount of time that must be allotted for this purpose. Evidence points to the fact that sleep is the logical time when all of the biological functions—including repair—take place at optimal efficiency. During this interval of rest, there is no strain or resistance of the musculature; circulation is working well; the liver function is not burdened by food that needs to be metabolized, so that waste-cleansing is more effective; and the colon muscles—no longer tense—can push the waste products along to their outlet. In brief, the relaxation allowed by sleep permits the body to function normally in every way, so that the biological processes take place in an unimpeded manner. It is precisely during this long rest period that the body has the energy and the ideal functional efficiency to do its greatest healing.

It is difficult to propose what any individual can do to encourage sleep or other forms of rest. All of us undoubtedly have our own strategies for getting ourselves into a mood for sleep. Sufficient exercise during the day, stress control procedures, and habituating ourselves to set periods for sleep are often helpful. What I can remind you of, however, is that the need for rest is always indicated by the body. It has its own language through which it communicates to us when it is in pain, or ill, and also when it needs rest.

Whenever it signals, we need to listen to our bodies. We don't necessarily believe that there exists a set cycle, like getting up at eight in the morning and going to bed at eleven in the evening. Some individuals have the kind of internal clock system that seems to work better when they go to bed at ten in the evening, or rise at four in the morning. Any time arrangement is suitable, so long as it provides enough sleep. And if you want to take a nap in the morning or afternoon as well, that's fine too.

Even at work you can use mid morning or afternoon breaks to put your head down on the desk, relax and shut your eyes for a spell. Or else, during the day you can usually find some quiet spot if you feel the need to rest. It is usually possible in all circumstances to take some time off from the day's activities—whether it is a short interval on the job, or a nap at home. This is the theme which I have tried to emphasize throughout this book: when you are dealing with your body's biological requirements, you try to find a way to serve those needs as well as you possibly can. Perhaps the book, *The Promise of Sleep*, about sleep deprivation by William Dement, M.D., might convince the reader that sleep is as important as food, air and water.

One of the ways in which the biological repair system differs from the traditional approach is that the patient is an active participant in the healing process, not simply a passive object who is acted upon by the doctor and his prescribed treatment modalities. For the most part, passive individuals do not become involved in biological therapies. Almost always, these therapies require judgement, effort and decision-making by the patient. The individual who prefers to place himself or herself totally in the hands of a doctor—one who gives drugs and other treatments and tells his patient exactly what to do—will end up with a conventional treatment.

Communication is, of course, a two-way avenue. Just as the doctor should not hold back vital information, the patient must learn to be open about his or her own feelings, reactions and misgivings. The patient should communicate these feelings clearly to the practitioner, keep him or her informed about symptoms and changes, and apply the repair procedures intelligently and without resistance. It is up to the patient to interpret what the body is saying, and to relate any significant signs that indicate that the biological therapy needs adjustment. Recovery will depend on the patient's active participation with the doctor. This partnership will provide the maximum opportunity for success.

9. Metabolic Programs and Adjunctive Therapies

Progress is impossible without change; and those who cannot change their minds cannot change anything.
—George Bernard Shaw

I resisted writing this chapter because therapies tend to change over time—sometimes there is an update in knowledge, sometimes essential supplies are no longer available, sometimes other programs are more efficient and provide better results, or there may be a variety of other reasons that would outdate material. The Board of Trustees of FACT and those working with me to prepare this book for publication urged me to include information about various therapies that I have acquired as president of FACT. I am doing this with some hesitation, as printed material sometimes survives beyond its authenticity.

In this chapter, I would like to discuss some of these alternative therapies, and some of the weaknesses and strengths of the various systems. I also want to make it clear that we at FACT support only those substances and techniques which are non-toxic and do no harm. Anything that is toxic or does harm will add to the burden of an already overtaxed system, and hamper the reversal of the health problem. The body's need to eliminate the accumulated toxins is already overtaxing its ability to reject material which it considers foreign. To add more toxic substances—even if they are labeled alternative—can only increase the difficulty of correcting the biological breakdown.

As we have already seen, even a small amount of poison taken consistently can contribute to the insidious process whereby toxins gradually build up over time and are stored in the cells, tissues and lymphatics. What sense does it make for an individual to use so-called alternatives, such as hydrazine sulfate, selenium, exaggerated amounts of vitamin C or any other biologically unsound substance or technique, when they will only interfere with the healing process?

I want to point out that it is not my purpose here to advise individuals on which specific substances or procedures to use. The choice of therapy is up to the person and his or her practitioner. It can only be made properly on the basis of the patient's particular health problems and needs. What I can do, however, is provide information and correct misinformation on different aspects of the various alternative therapies with which I have had considerable experience. This material has been made available to the public through our magazine, *Cancer Forum*, and in other printed matter.

I have acquired extensive knowledge on this subject; and yet, with all of my considerable expertise, it would be unwise to claim to be on target one hundred percent of the time. One can therefore imagine what can happen when untrained or amateur individuals disseminate information about alternatives that are inappropriate, untested, produce meager results, or may be harmful. Cancer patients must be extremely cautious before they choose any particular therapy.

Hopefully, the material in this chapter will provide the reader with a better understanding of the potential and limitation of some of the therapies. Once the person is in possession of some facts, he or she will be in a position to make more informed decisions on which therapy is best suited to his or her own specific needs.

METABOLIC PROGRAMS

Nutrition is such an integral part of restoring health—as cells are made of the food we ingest. It probably would be negligent if the metabolic programs were not given priority consideration and ample space in these pages. Nutrition is the primary tool to restore the body's ability to produce healthy cells and restore and maintain strong immune function.

I should add here that there is no quick or easy way to master a nutritional approach. Although the concept is simple to understand, the system requires experience and knowledge. I know a doctor, who, when he decided to learn nutrition properly, took a sabbatical to accomplish this. It is the logical way to acquire in-depth knowledge about metabolic systems. As I have pointed out, medical schools do not provide much nutritional instruction. The limited hours that schools devote to this subject are not nearly sufficient for one to become proficient in nutritional counseling. I understand, however, that some medical institutions are beginning to develop better nutritional curriculums.

Though I have previously emphasized the prime importance of nutrition in effecting biorepairs, I feel that there are a number of dietary programs that merit special attention due to the good results they have achieved.

The Gerson Therapy

The clinical and research work of Dr. Max Gerson is, without a doubt, the best documented biological program available. Most of the patients who sought his help were terminally ill or were told that there was no more that could be done for them. Others who went to him for treatment remained on their conventional regimes because of their fear of adopting a system that was not embraced by the medical establishment. Unfortunately, radiation and chemotherapy, because they are harmful, handicap the restoration capability of a biorepair system. Therefore, these patients were not the ideal subjects for repair. In his book, *A Cancer Therapy: Results of Fifty Cases*, Dr. Gerson presented 50 recovered patients, documenting his clinical activities and the different aspects of his approach. Forty-eight of these patients had been on conventional protocols when they came to him; two were not, and one of those was a trusting relative. Fortunately, the orthodox programs (especially chemotherapy) of his day were not quite as destructive to the host as they are today. Since the damage to the patient was not too extreme, it still was possible for the body to effect a repair. Today's aggressive use of chemotherapy and radiation all too often compromise the repair capability of the organism beyond reversal. When Dr. Gerson's book was written, about 1958, his cure rate, which included difficult cases, was about thirty-five percent—a very good track record. Ultimately, he did even better, but these later cases were not added to the book.

Dr. Gerson had unusual success with many types of cancer—including brain tumor, melanoma, breast cancer, uterine, etc. Metabolic healing methods are nonspecific, as the focus is not aimed at reducing the tumor's size, but on restoring the body's ability to metabolize food efficiently in order to produce healthy cells and to enhance immune activity. A healthy immune system will seek out abnormal cells as foreign substances and eliminate them.

One 88-year-old woman, still spry and healthy, who had been treated by Dr. Gerson 22 years earlier, approached me at a convention telling me how Dr. Gerson had saved and prolonged her life. Remember that he had his practice in the 1940s and 1950s, and this meeting took place in the early eighties. For cancer patients, particularly those very ill, that is an extraordinary record.

Dr. Gerson, who died in 1959, began his work in Germany during the time of Hitler. He came to New York City, started his program at Gotham Hospital, but found that he couldn't control the diet he had designed for his patients. Orderlies, nurses and visitors brought them junk foods after hours because the patients were unhappy with the more restricted, restorative dietary regimens he had arranged for them. Consequently, he set up his own clinic in Nanuet, New York, where eventually he became so overwhelmed with work, his wife had to protect him and turn away many patients. Some were brought on stretchers and deposited on his doorstep—he would always try, somehow, to help them. But if he discovered that a patient was not adhering to his program—and he could tell by measuring responses—he discouraged them from continuing as his patient. Many patients have a tendency to incorporate ideas that appear in health publications, books, radio talks, lectures and even suggestions from other patients, which have no applicability to their own condition. This pattern of behavior will sabotage a carefully-designed, metabolic program by causing an imbalance and creating confusion in measuring the patient's progress.

Dr. Gerson's program was a carefully developed nutritional regime that omitted all fats and oils from the diet for a period of time—except for flax-seed oil, which was included to obtain the essential fatty acids. Everything possible was done not to stress the liver. Dr. Gerson attached great importance to the liver's role in curing the patient, as this organ is responsible for a host of vital functions, including metabolism and detoxification. By controlling oils and fats, he gave the liver a chance to rest and restore in order to perform its normal functions. If there was less than about 30% liver function remaining, the doctor avoided taking the patient in the belief that it was too late to reverse the liver degeneration to effect recovery.

Dr. Gerson tells a story on a tape I have of a lecture he gave to a group of doctors at Dr. Bernard Jensen's Hidden Valley Health Ranch in Escondido, California. It is about a family that brought their elderly mother to him for treatment. He found that her liver was in bad shape, so he felt he could not cure her so refused to accept her for treatment. Nevertheless, despite his reluctance, the family left her with him. His program was able to restore her energy, albeit, temporarily. She survived comfortably for a year and a half, but the liver continued to deteriorate as he expected and it was this loss of liver function that finally caused her demise.

As part of Dr. Gerson's protocol, he included the use of thyroid substance, lugol solution, and other items as indicated. These were added under careful supervision. The juices that were part of the regime included a measured amount of potassium of which patients had to drink an exact amount every day. He also used liver juice. Because of the difficulty in obtaining unpolluted livers from organically-fed animals at the present time, the Gerson Institute program in Mexico has been revised and other liver support materials have been substituted.

An integral aspect of the Gerson program—a practice which he developed and perfected—was the coffee enema. Its inclusion in the restoration system was based on scientific research which had been done by Kaspar Blond. Before I discuss this, I want to point out some of the hazards of using *any retention enema* without knowledge of the physiology of a rectal infusion. There are too many people who assume that the coffee enema constituted the major part of the Gerson program, and that this particular technique was the single system that accomplished the cure. Suggestions to use coffee enemas are often proposed from platforms, or written about in "natural health" books by well-meaning people who are genuinely trying to help others, but lack adequate experience—a hazardous practice.

What one should be aware of is that a coffee enema (retention enema) requires holding the infusion for about 15 minutes to effect absorption. The purpose of the coffee enema is for the caffeine in the coffee to be absorbed by the portal vein to stimulate bile flow from the liver. If an individual has toxic wastes in the colon, and holds liquid in the colon, it will begin to dissolve some of those toxic by-products which have been stored in that area. Understandably, if toxic wastes are dissolved in the colon, they are going to be absorbed back into the bloodstream with the caffeine. The last thing to be desired is for the toxins to be redeposited in the bloodstream and recirculated through the liver. If this should happen repeatedly, the liver—and sometimes the adrenals as well—will become exhausted in the process. That is why having clinic experience and understanding the physiology of the particular methods are crucial before applying some of these therapeutic systems.

The Gerson program is primarily a vegetarian system. From my years of experience with patients and clinicians, I feel, although this is a good system, the results could be improved if the system was adjusted for those individuals who *need meat for metabolic balance*. Research has shown that some cancer patients are meat metabolizers and need meat protein in their diet in order to build good quality cells. In actuality, Dr. Gerson did not have a total vegetarian program; it only seemed so. He used meat in the form of liver juice. Since it is very difficult to obtain uncontaminated, organic livers, it had to be eliminated from the original system and another form of organic meat protein should be substituted. Another change that would make this system more feasible without altering its efficacy is to substitute barberry for the coffee enema. Barberry is an herb that stimulates bile flow, just the same as what is accomplished with the caffeine. (Nature usually produces more than one element to provide the same function.) It would also eliminate the risk of dissolved colon toxins being recirculated, and make it easier to continue the program after leaving the clinic. This is a labor-intensive system. While at the clinic, the work is done by the staff. At home, it becomes difficult for some people to continue carrying out this heavy program without help, so some people unfortunately discontinue it out of necessity. I am sure it could be modified for home use.

The Kelley Metabolic Program

The Kelley Metabolic Program is a dietary regime created by Dr. William D. Kelley, largely as a consequence of service that he received as a cancer patient himself under the guidance of Dr. Howard Beard of Fort Worth, Texas. It is actually an adaptation of different dietary systems carefully put together into a workable regimen that has been effective for a large number of patients. I have probably had contact with more individuals on this regime than any of the other biological programs. Years ago, when FACT first began its work and got positive feedback about Kelley's program, we arranged a system whereby one individual carried blood samples for a group of ten people to Dr. Kelley's office, which was then located in Grapevine, Texas. Analyses of the samples would come back to FACT in the form of audio tapes for distribution to the patients' doctors. By listening to the tapes, we could hear for ourselves what their metabolic program was and follow the patient's progress. All of the patients were under the care of their individual physicians, as this was one of Kelley's requirements for people interested in the program.

In Kelley's program, patients are evaluated to determine their individual physiological weaknesses. The regime is then designed to address the patient's requirements. They are put on a diet of juices, mostly raw foods, some cooked foods, and supplementary materials, consisting of mainly enzymes and glandulars. These supplements are designed, not haphazardly, but in accordance with the patient's physiological needs. Dr. Kelley placed a great deal of emphasis on the use of pancreatic enzymes, in higher doses than needed, just for protein metabolism. His program depends upon these enzymes to destroy the cancer cells. His reasoning is that cancer cells are essentially protein and therefore the patient needs the pancreatic enzymes to digest and metabolize the excess amount of protein.

As previously stated, the excess protein that some people eat is stored on the periphery of cells, where it may become dense enough to prevent the cells from getting sufficient nutrients and oxygen. In the light of this research, you can understand the value of pancreatic enzymes. I should add that Dr. Kelley's program is suitable for other degenerative health problems, as it reestablishes homeostasis. As with all successful programs, detoxification is emphasized and an appropriate method is incorporated into the system.

The Waerland System

The Waerland system, which is available in many clinics in Europe, is carefully designed so that every component serves a specific purpose. Patients start out in the morning with a broth of cooked potatoes and other vegetables, and the alkaline drink Excelsior. According to the Waerland philosophy, healing takes place mostly during the night, when sleep allows the energy to be shifted into the healing phase, whereas, during the waking hours, most of our energy is used for eating, metabolism, walking and a host of other activities. Because healing takes place when the body is at rest, in the morning the individual's bloodstream is heavily laden with the toxins the cells have discarded. These wastes can have a deleterious effect if allowed to remain in the patient's bloodstream. It is therefore necessary to neutralize and eliminate these acidic toxins before one takes the first daily meal at breakfast. Excelsior, an alkaline broth, is considered to be the best way to give the body the required alkaline mineral salts to perform this detoxification task.

The usual routine for the patients is to have a fruit breakfast, to which can be added yogurt or clabbered milk. The yogurt or clabbered milk replaces the "friendly" intestinal flora which the body requires. These bacteria tend to be washed away by the enemas which are part of the Waerland system.

Lunch and dinner menus are interchangeable. There is usually a large raw salad. Raw food is used by all good metabolic programs to provide patients with the intrinsic factors in unheated food that are essential for healing and normal cell production. This is also the source for the alkalinity that is essential to establish a balanced program. It is abundant in greens and other raw vegetables. It is, of course, essential that the body get both alkaline and acid foods in the correct balance, but the acid quota is much smaller than alkaline. Ideally, 20% of our intake must be acid; it can be higher but not greater than the intake of alkaline food. Some natural healers advocate 80% alkaline and 20% acid. It doesn't have to be that exact, but alkaline must be over 50% of the total intake.

The typical diet for most people today consists of large portions of meat, fish, eggs and other acid foods. At the Waerland Clinics these foods are omitted from the diet, and raw foods, vegetable juices and herbal teas are encouraged. As you can see, it is a vegetarian diet (which may not be suitable for everyone). The protein supply consists mainly of nuts, some beans and a small amount of cheese and clabbered milk. A liquid fast with raw vegetable juices diluted with distilled water, herbal teas, broth and other liquids is the Waerland detoxification system. To further aid in eliminating toxic body wastes, enemas are required, as well as physical exercise, plenty of fresh air, baths and skin brushing to maintain open pores. A proper mental attitude is also considered important in the recovery process.

According to Dr. Karl Aly, retired administrator of Tallmogarden, a 90-bed clinic in Sweden which uses the Waerland dietary system, supplementary materials such as herbals, natural vitamins, as well as other nontoxic elements are sometimes given to the patients to stimulate the immune system and cell metabolism.

The Wigmore Program

The Wigmore Program is best known for its use of wheat grass juice and sprouts. These are some of the biological materials used as part of an overall dietary and detoxification regime. For those individuals who are able to stay at one of the Ann Wigmore Centers, the program can be put into effect in its totality. There, patients are placed on a raw food dietary program, which includes wheat grass and sprouts as well as a full nutritional regimen. Wheat grass, when juiced, is claimed to contain all of the components of the bloodstream, so that it serves as a quite nourishing overall component of the program. However, by itself, wheat grass is not to be considered a complete form of therapy.

The Wigmore program is a very useful therapy and has the advantage of not being exorbitant in cost. However, the complication with this program arises when the patient returns home, especially in a northern climate and to a city apartment which does not have enough room or sun to grow the wheat grass in sufficient amounts for juicing. Eydie May Hunsberger, author of *How I Conquered Cancer Naturally*, about her successful experience with breast cancer on the Wigmore program, lived on a ranch in Southern California, where she built a greenhouse for growing the amount of wheat grass needed for juicing. Therefore, growing her supply was possible in summer and winter. Since it might be difficult for some patients to continue this program after the initial stay at the center, one can benefit by starting at the center and then shifting to another metabolic regimen that is more practical to follow at home. There is a wheat grass supplement now available in health food stores. However, it is difficult to determine if it can serve as a substitute for the fresh juice.

The Work of Dr. Norman Walker

While we are on the subject of quality dietary regimes, we cannot ignore the work of Dr. Norman W. Walker. He died at the age of 117 quietly in his sleep. Many people consider him the dean of the natural health movement. Before he retired to Phoenix, Arizona, he had an active clinical practice in New Jersey. His ideas, which were carefully gathered over many decades of experience with cancer and other health problems, are available in the many books he authored. His books are still being published, as they provide basic understanding of the value and uses of foods in a way that is different from most other nutritional books. They are considered classics in the health field.

Dr. Walker was a vegetarian who ate only raw foods plus cheese. As we now know, not everyone can get along on the total vegetarian diet, as some people need small quantities of flesh foods. This is probably due to the fact that after generations of meat-eating ancestors, our bodies have adapted to our environment—another example of Nature's wisdom. But for those who can get along with this vegetarian, nutritional regime, it can be a very beneficial program.

The first vegetable juice extractor was developed by Dr. Walker. It is still being sold today—the Norwalk juicer. Laboratory tests show that it extracts a wide range of elements from vegetables and fruits. It also extracts a large quantity of juice from carrots, which is evident in a very dry pulp.

The Work of Dr. Bernard Jensen

Dr. Jensen was the foremost authority in iris analysis and was known worldwide for his expertise in this field. His nutritional knowledge was based on six decades of clinic work at the Hidden Valley Health Ranch, which he owned and directed, in Escondido, California. Through his vast experience as a practitioner, he helped scores of individuals with his carefully conceived and biologically-oriented programs.

Dr. Jensen developed prostate cancer in his late eighties, probably due to his extensive travelling to frequent lectures. His food intake on these lecture tours was not what he was accustomed to and not always wholesome. Constant adjustment to unfamiliar conditions automatically puts an enormous strain on the body. He was able to correct the prostate condition and continued, until his recent death, to lead a vigorous life at an age when most people would consider retirement. His restoration system included a metabolic program, exercise, detoxification, relaxation, careful supplementation, as well as addressing any and all physiological essentials. Dr. Jensen was an early advocate for using a slant board to improve circulation and a bouncer to pump the lymphatics.

He adopted some of the beneficial aspects of the Waerland system, such as his own version of Excelsior, the alkaline broth. He also created his version of the Waerland cereal—Thermos-cooked cereal which uses whole grains prepared so as not to destroy their natural enzymes. It is important to understand why grains are one of the valuable components of a healthy program. Just visualize each seed when it is put in the soil and watered; it will grow into a new plant with all of its life-giving energy. Because it also produces new seeds, it has to have balanced hormones. Grains are, therefore, an excellent source of natural hormones and may help those needing balanced hormones to correct osteoporosis. See page 99 for more information on preparing this whole grain cereal.

ADJUNCTIVE THERAPIES

Over the years, FACT has had considerable experience with cancer patients who have utilized a number of supplementary procedures and substances in addition to those we have already discussed in these pages. I have found, from my contact with patients and practitioners, that these adjunctive therapies can, under certain circumstances, be excellent aids in boosting the body's healing capability.

There are, for example, a number of substances such as the Hoxsey Herbal Tonic, Iscador, Essiac, and others which come under the heading of botanicals. These herbs can sometimes help the system loosen up and remove toxins, as well as stimulate circulation, liver function and glandular activity. However, it is important to remember that there is no magic potion, as a total biological repair of body chemistry is necessary.

People collect a lot of information about a particular substance—whether it is Laetrile, Essiac, Shark Cartilage, Carnivora, Hoxsey, Selenium, Iscador, etc.—and think all they have to do is get this magic potion, get the proper injections, do as the doctor orders, and they are well on their way to recovery. I could go through all of the therapies, and there are many, and make the same comment: "They do not address the breakdown in body chemistry and cell production."

There are also treatments such as cell therapy, immunotherapy and fever therapy which can provide the body with a valuable boost in its effort toward recovery. I am not minimizing the value of these biological alternative therapies when they are applied under the proper supervision as part of an overall repair regime. I have, for instance, seen a number of cases where immunotherapy has helped to strengthen the body's defense system much faster than a metabolic program alone. So, too, cellular therapy has shown itself to be a useful tool in assisting the body to make a biological repair faster than nutrition alone. I have already related several instances where fever therapy (systemic thermotherapy) has helped reduce the tumor without harm to the patient.

It should be emphasized, however, that none of these supplementary therapies provide the needed vitamins, minerals, enzymes, complex carbohydrates (starches), essential fatty acids, etc. that are needed to correct cell production; therefore, they cannot be considered a definitive cure for cancer without a metabolic program. They are good adjunctives, but they do not address the basic problem of the need for rebalancing body chemistry and correcting the vital role of cell production.

I believe—and this is the overriding theme of this book—that the best way to treat cancer is by treating the host. Unless the breakdown in body chemistry, which I consider responsible for producing abnormal cells, is repaired, any supplemental substance or technique is going to provide only limited usefulness. There is every probability that the cancer will occur again and again in a body that is not wholly repaired. This concept applies regardless of the therapy used and to alternative as well as traditional methods.

In virtually every situation that I know of where an adjunctive therapy was successful to the extent where the patient was able to regain his or her health over the long term, that individual was on a biologically-sound repair program. This included a metabolic regime as well as detoxification procedures to rid the body of accumulated toxins that helped create the illness in the first place. In addition, attention was paid to other areas in need of correction, such as structural alignment; or the control of nervous tension through massage, biofeedback, or other techniques that control stress. When the different aspects of the cancer patient's biological deficiencies and dysfunctions are being dealt with, a safe adjunctive therapy can provide the body with additional help on the pathway to repair.

Immunotherapy

At one time immunotherapy was a stranger to the cancer scene. Antonio Rottino, M.D., head of Hodgkin's disease research at St. Vincent's Hospital in New York City, concluded that there was a connection between immunity and cancer long before the establishment accepted the link. An immunity link to cancer, at that time, was unheard of so it was considered somewhat strange. Two of his assistants, Dr. Lawrence Burton and Dr. Frank Friedman, decided to expand on the immunity concept and branched out on their own. Ultimately, Dr. Friedman quit, but Burton continued the immunity work in Great Neck, New York. Because of the hostile nature of the medical community, he eventually left the United States to settle in the Bahamas.

Dr. Burton's type of immunotherapy is quite complex. Patients have to travel to the clinic, be evaluated for immune competence, have their immune substance formulated, then go home and continue the program under the guidance of the clinic. In many instances it requires as many as 12 injections per day and this goes on for an extended period of time.

Today, immunotherapy is accepted and available at many clinics in the United States. It is no longer considered unusual even though it is not yet a routine therapy. Some confusion still exists about immune enhancement (sometimes referred to as immune modulation) at the clinics in this country because the physiology of activating the immune system is not understood as well as it should be. An active immune system will use its energy to do what it does naturally—reject any foreign material—and it considers cancer cells foreign.

An active immune system will start what I refer to as a "house cleaning." Stored toxins will be released uncontrollably from the storage areas and flood the bloodstream, causing severe to mild autointoxication. A knowledgeable immunotherapist, who recognizes and understands the symptoms, can control the pace of activity and avoid any discomfort or risk. The immune substance itself is not toxic, as some practitioners assume. The toxic symptoms come from the movement of the toxins from storage, which usually generates fever or flu symptoms. Fever is Nature's healing mechanism.

Whole–Body Hyperthermia

I have touched on this therapy in an earlier chapter. It is variously called whole-body hyperthermia, systemic thermotherapy, fever therapy and other terms used to signify raising body temperature. Heat therapy has been used for centuries as a method of treating many different forms of disease. The concept of raising body temperature for fighting cancer was started in Germany, but used by a limited group of centers. Eventually, Dr. Robert Pettigrew of Scotland began research by immersing patients in a melted wax bath to maintain a temperature of 110°F which he achieved by pumping hot air through the patient's mouth. He reported very impressive results.

About 25 years ago I learned of the work here in the United States of Robert Berman, M.D., at St. John's Hospital in Far Rockaway, NY. He developed water-filled blankets which were heated to raise the patient's body temperature. The blankets made the process of hyperthermia more efficient. Ultimately, I found an oncologist, Dr. Donald Cole and his colleague, Dr. John Pung, who were interested in this unusual (at that time) system. Dr. Cole's interest was piqued because his mother, a lymphoma patient, developed a spontaneous fever and survived for twenty years. Dr. Berman loaned Dr. Cole and Dr. Pung his equipment and taught them the technique. Their work produced very positive results in tumor reduction in patients who were good candidates for the procedure. (Patients with weak hearts cannot tolerate the high temperature of 107°F and patients with poor kidney function cannot eliminate the dead cancer cells adequately.)

The National Cancer Institute launched a hyperthermia research project under the guidance of Joan Bull, M.D. Although she treated only advanced cancer patients who were no longer offered available treatment, the results were quite successful in terms of restoring the patient's well-being, actual tumor destruction and additional quality time. Some patients who had previously been addicted to narcotics, because of extreme pain, became pain-free after the heat therapy.

The potential for this treatment appears to be excellent. It is essentially a non-lethal, non-mutilating procedure which can be used in conjunction with, or subsequent to, other forms of biological therapy, such as a metabolic program. It is *especially useful* for patients who have failed to improve their condition on any therapy or where other treatments are inappropriate.

There are two forms of heat therapy. Some groups have adopted a technique of local hyperthermia, using microwaves or radio waves to generate heat. In my opinion, a local effect in which only the tumor is treated does not solve the problem, since cancer is a generalized disease. Whole-body hyperthermia, which duplicates Nature's design, encompasses the entire body and destroys any micrometastases, which have probably not been clinically detected.

This non-toxic procedure should be an accepted, routine part of the cancer protocol. It should be a first choice before radiation or chemotherapy and possibly, in some instances even before surgery. Unfortunately, the Food and Drug Administration has labeled whole-body hyperthermia experimental—even though it has been used for years with thousands of patients and heat is known unequivocally to destroy cancer cells. The experimental category relieves insurance carriers from including it as a third-party-payer. I believe if a trial were run to compare costs, it would show that hyperthermia is cost effective, which would please the insurance industry. I am quite certain that if medical insurance covered systemic hyperthermia, it would be available routinely, as medical institutions prefer to rely on payment from insurance companies.

Botanicals

Botanicals, or herbals, as they are more commonly called, have been used by natural healers for years and have proven to be effective in many ways. They can support the healing process when used competently, without the side effects usually associated with most of the pharmaceuticals. Since "do no harm" is the yardstick, the herbals are wonderful resources for relief of troublesome symptoms.

Hoxsey Herbal Therapy

This therapy uses an herbal tonic consisting of a combination of ten specially prepared herbs which are distributed by the Bio-Medical Center, a clinic in Tijuana, Mexico. The doctors at the clinic do a thorough physical examination to determine the quantity of material that is appropriate for each patient. In some instances a special formula may be created if there is an unusual problem. The therapy also includes a nutritional regimen which is not as optimum as FACT's standard or those designed by practitioners who specialize in metabolic therapies. That doesn't create a problem as the dietary program can be improved.

The system was developed by Harry Hoxsey, a veterinarian, who observed horses recover from sickness by selecting certain herbs from the array that grew naturally where the animals grazed. Harry Hoxsey wrote a book entitled *You Don't Have to Die* about his therapy and his struggle with the medical authorities. The antagonism of the past against anything other than the conventional protocols of radiation, chemotherapy or surgery seems to have subsided considerably. Herbs have received a new status in the medical community to the extent that there is now a *Physicians' Desk Reference for Herbal Medicine*.

Essiac

Rene Caisse, a Canadian nurse, developed the herbal formula Essiac (which represents her name in reverse). Essiac contains four primary herbs: slippery elm inner bark, burdock root, sheep sorrel, and Indian rhubarb root. The combination of these herbs can help restore body chemistry through the cleansing and elimination of toxins.

Working as a nurse in Canada, Rene Caisse and a group of medical associates experimented with mice and perfected the tonic. Doctors began to refer their terminal cases to her and the results were unusually good. In 1938, she applied to parliament for recognition of the formula and lost by only three votes. In the years since then, it has been used with documentation of safety and effectiveness on thousands of humans in clinics and by doctors in both the United States and Canada.

She gave it to one group only—the Resperin Corporation—because she felt the Resperin board members had the proper credentials and government connections to prod the Canadian agency responsible for authorizing official testing of Essiac, to do so. Since Rene Caisse is no longer living, anyone can claim they have the formula; there is no one to discredit the claim.

There are, no doubt, differences in the potency of the formula as it is prepared today because it is no longer prescribed in the same dose that Rene Caisse used. The suggested dose today is to drink more than one cup of Essiac tea daily. When Rene Caisse gave the tonic to patients, she suggested using a cup as seldom as twice a week. In instances when the cancer was more advanced, she would recommend a daily cupful. This is quite a bit less than the amount that Resperin Corporation now suggests.

Cellular Therapy

Cellular therapy is a technique in which suspended and specially prepared animal fetal organ cells are injected intramuscularly into the patient to *rejuvenate degenerated or weak organs.* To my knowledge, this procedure was first discovered and applied by a Dr. Keuttner in 1912, but it was eventually forgotten. In 1931, Dr. Paul Niehans, who became interested in cell therapy because of Dr. Keuttner's work, reintroduced the method when he was asked to treat an emergency patient after her parathyroids were accidentally injured during surgery at a nearby hospital. He was raising black lambs so he took the parathyroid glands from the fetus of a pregnant animal, chopped it crudely and put it into a syringe. This was then injected into the patient. The healthy animal cells were accepted automatically by the related gland, the parathyroids, and the patient recovered, which was most unusual. Ultimately, Dr. Niehans opened a clinic in Montreux,

Switzerland, called La Prairie; it is still doing cellular therapy today, primarily to reverse the aging process.

At first, this technique, which is called fresh-cell therapy, made it imperative that the cell sample be from a freshly-killed donor animal, selected properly, assured of sterility, and injected into the recipient in as short a time as possible. In about 1951, a dry-cell method was perfected and is still in use today. Tissue samples are collected and quickly freeze-dried for later use. These lyophilized cells can be stored for a long time and will maintain their full potency.

In spite of all the research, the mechanism by which cell therapy works is considered elusive by some practitioners. Science and medicine are so bogged down in research formats that even when a system is obvious, they hesitate coming to a definitive conclusion. The orthodox medical community fears being challenged if a procedure doesn't fulfil the established method of complex, conclusive research. The standard of judgement is not necessarily applicable to biological systems of healing. Natural processes need not be evaluated by the same standards used for testing toxic chemicals.

There is a natural affinity for the implanted cells to seek out their own kind, be adopted by the related organ and thus cause the organ to displace the weaker cells. Since the bloodstream collects the discarded cells to be processed for elimination, the bloodstream temporarily becomes toxic. This toxicity cannot be ignored. Experienced cell therapists usually have a detoxification method in place for use both before and after the procedure.

The effect of cell therapy is to rehabilitate or rejuvenate. This strengthens the biological activity of the organ or organ groups at which the cellular therapy is aimed. Therefore cellular therapy can produce quite lasting effects if a wholesome lifestyle is subsequently adopted. Returning to the same lifestyle responsible for the original breakdown will eventually cause the same breakdown of cells in the organs which were rejuvenated.

According to Dr. Anthony Schenk, a specialist in cell therapy who frequently addressed the annual FACT convention, cellular therapy is applicable to precancerous as well as cancer-stricken patients, and postoperative cases. Although it is inconclusive, there seems to be some indication that cellular therapy can serve as a preventive measure by strengthening host resistance. Dr. Schenk points out that cellular therapy is indicated not only for cancer, but wherever there is a disturbance in the biological process which can lead to chronic degenerative failure of adequate body function.

"We are convinced," he notes, "that cellular therapy is a very important weapon in the field of medical therapy; and very often, when everything else fails or when there is no other way to go, it is effective."

FACT does not consider cellular therapy a total treatment by itself, but it can be an invaluable part of the process of restoring body chemistry to its optimum function. A revitalized body will then be capable of processing its nutrients for competent production of healthy cells and eliminating toxic accumulation. This restoration will in turn strengthen the patient's defense system.

Stem Cells

After 70 years of cell therapy use in Europe, Canada, Mexico and other places outside of our country, there is a great hubbub of interest and research taking place now in the United States regarding stem cells. It is the new frontier and an advanced type of cell therapy. Stem cells are derived from the umbilical cord blood and the placenta, which provides an abundant supply of high quality undifferentiated cells. This technique eliminates the need to slaughter animals or use embryonic cells from abortions, which generates religious controversy. The scope of what stem cells can do, in a vast number of degenerative problems and in accident cases where nerves are damaged, may seem like a medical miracle.

Clinical work on stem cells is as yet too limited for statistical evaluations of posttreatment effectiveness. Nevertheless, using the information from long years of research and clinical work in cellular therapy as a guide, it is my belief that stem cells should be available as rapidly as possible. Otherwise, many people who could benefit greatly will be deprived of this excellent source for healing.

This new development is creating new industries. Some sources are not only suggesting that the umbilical cord and the placenta be frozen for future use but it has already been done in many instances. In most of the cell therapy clinics in Europe, cells are freeze-dried to preserve them. Possibly the pharmaceutical industry in the United States might eventually evaluate the same process. I would assume that lyophilizing the placenta, umbilical cord, and cord blood cells would preserve them as well and make them more readily available to the medical profession. (It is interesting to note that Adan Graetz, M.D. suggested storing amniotic fluid when he investigated and developed its use while interning at the Women's Hospital of the University of Zurich as early as 1965.)

There are a myriad of other so-called alternative cancer therapies that I am deliberately not writing about because they are not relevant to the *concept of restoring homeostasis as presented in this book.* Since repairing and restoring health is the thrust of this publication, we need to differentiate between those therapies called alternatives that enhance a patient's well-being, and those that duplicate the medical model of treatment which concentrates on tumor destruction, or is toxic, or simply mediocre. A therapy labelled alternative, based on the principle of blocking nourishment to the cell causing it to die, is a typical concept of traditional chemotherapy. Unfortunately, it also will cause the death of healthy cells, as chemotherapy cannot be selective. The goal should be to protect the integrity of the body by following Hippocrates' admonition of doing no harm, so that the body retains its ability to repair. The healthy cell destruction of conventional chemotherapy ultimately takes a heavy toll on the well-being of the host—too often precluding a full repair.

There are about eighty therapies called alternatives *that are not alternative in concept.* Some are called alternative only because they are not sanctioned by officialdom. It is important to remember that that does not automatically translate into a therapy that produces the positive long-term results that are the true goal of the cancer patient.

Appendix I: Case Histories

Until man duplicates a blade of grass,
Nature can laugh at his so-called scientific knowledge.
—THOMAS ALVA EDISON

From time to time, FACT publishes the experiences of cancer patients who regained their health as a result of their involvement in a biorepair program. It is done in the belief that making their stories public in the pages of our magazine, *Cancer Forum,* will provide helpful information on different aspects of biological therapies for people who are interested in alternative approaches to cancer. The case histories I have chosen for inclusion in this chapter exemplify the most basic components of any sound repair system—nutrition and detoxification.

In my view, an individual is not considered to have recovered simply because the *major* symptom of cancer, the tumor, has been removed or reduced, whether by surgery, chemotherapy, radiation or any other form of therapy. The mere disappearance of the tumor, even up to the five-year survival period which is considered a "cure" in conventional medicine, is by no means an indication that the patient's health problem has been resolved. Excising the malignant mass may bring an interval of reprieve, but it will not of itself repair the biological dysfunction that led to the development of abnormal cells. As I have tried to demonstrate, cancer affects not one single organ alone, but the human system in general. Consequently, the restoration of health can take place only when the biological breakdown has been repaired, whether spontaneously or through diligent effort, by rebalancing the entire system and correcting the biochemical breakdown. This concept is applicable to conventional as well as alternative therapies.

Before FACT makes a public presentation of a patient's case history, we have to be sure there is medical evidence, such as x-rays and biopsy, to confirm that the cancerous condition did in fact exist. In addition, the patient would have to be on a biorepair regimen—which of course is the use of non-toxic forms of therapy. Finally, an interval of at least ten years should have passed before the patient can be considered recovered. We at FACT have very exacting criteria for evaluating a so-called recovery. In comparing it to a similar situation of someone on conventional therapy, it has to be evident that the biological repair has benefited the individual significantly on a long-term basis. As much as is possible, we keep in close touch with patients to check on their progress and to provide any information that may be required.

"Cancer Need Not Be Fatal"

Pat Judson

Pat Judson was the former president of the now discontinued Metro-Detroit Chapter of FACT. Over thirty years ago she was sent home by a doctor who told her that there was nothing more that conventional medicine could do to alleviate her cancer. This sentence of doom came after she had received medical treatment for several years for colitis and then was operated on for cancer of the colon. One of the doctors who performed the surgery told Mrs. Judson that she had the fastest-growing type of cancer known to medicine. It was his opinion that neither cobalt (a type of radiation) nor chemotherapy could help her. Expressing surprise that she had even survived the surgical procedure, he informed her that in his opinion she had about six months to a year to live. Despite the apparent hopelessness of her condition, she was given diethylstilbestrol (DES) for hormone balance, since they had also removed her ovaries.

The surgeon's prediction notwithstanding, Mrs. Judson lived past the time that had been allotted her. In January 1972, almost two years after the original surgery, she experienced a recurrence of the blockage in the colon. Fearful that her surgeon would immediately hospitalize her if she went to him for advice, she found what she considered to be a more understanding doctor. After he treated her to the best of his ability, he told her that she would have to return to her doctor for surgery. It was his opinion that she could not live much longer if she refused, since her cancer had spread to the lymph glands. When she asked him how long he believed she could survive after surgery, he expressed strong doubts that he could be of any great help and gave her possibly up to three months.

After considerable thought and discussion with her family, she decided she could not endure another surgical ordeal. Instead, she chose what she thought was certain death and trusted without question the judgement of the doctors who had said that nothing could be done to cure her. There was, however, a quality in Pat's makeup that would not allow her to accept passively the certainty of death. It was, as she termed it, "an inner voice" telling her that death need not be the inevitable fate of the cancer victim.

Shortly afterwards, she learned about a metabolic program guided by Dr. William D. Kelley. He had been restoring cancer patients to health by means of a system of nutritional and other biological therapies that he had developed in the course of overcoming his own cancer.

Mrs. Judson visited Dr. Kelley in January of 1972. She spent a full day in his office for an evaluation of her weaknesses in order for him to design an individualized metabolic program that addressed her specific breakdown. He determined from a blood sample, which he then subjected to a computer analysis, that she had a critically high cancer index. On the basis of this analysis, and a thorough examination of her life and health patterns, he devised a regimen of improved nutrition, rest, exercise and detoxification. Making no promises that she would be cured of cancer, he merely told her to follow faithfully and intelligently the program he had prescribed, and to return in six months.

For about five months after this first visit, Mrs. Judson followed this vigorous program, which required a complete change in her lifestyle. It also entailed major alterations in the way in which her family lived, so that they could understand the basic principals of her metabolic regime and support her knowledgeably in carrying out her nutritional and other programs.

She gradually became accustomed to a daily routine of enemas, sitz baths, sweat baths to help her cleanse her system, long walks for exercise, and plenty of sleep and rest to give her body an opportunity to heal.

Following Dr. Kelley's instructions, she eliminated from her diet certain foods and drinks, such as: coffee, tea, alcoholic beverages and soft drinks. She also omitted sugar, white flour and other devitalized foods. Her new nutritional regime, aimed at substituting high-quality nutrients for the unwholesome foods she had been eating up until then, consisted mainly of raw vegetables and vegetable juice, fresh fruits, protein, soaked raw grains, nuts, complex carbohydrates, as well as carefully selected food supplements that were applicable to her physiological needs.

When she returned to Dr. Kelley for an examination, his tests revealed that her cancer index had dropped to within the range that was considered normal. Not only did it appear that her cancer was now under control diagnostically, but she felt better than at any previous period in her life, even before the onset of her illness. Today, approximately thirty years after being told by her doctors that her condition was hopeless and only drugs could provide pain relief, she is in good health.

An interesting sidelight of her story is that on her second visit to Dr. Kelley, she brought along all of her family to be checked out. Among the family was a daughter of ten who, at the time, was falling backward in school. After Dr. Kelley put the child on a balanced nutritional program, she began to make such rapid progress in her studies that her teachers were amazed. Before Mrs. Judson's discovery that nutrition could bring about mental as well as physical benefits, she and her family had experienced many agonizing hours with doctors and school personnel attempting unsuccessfully to help her daughter succeed.

"Eating to Live, Not Living to Eat"

Richard A. Mott:

In June of 1972 Richard Mott, who had been feeling increasingly ill and short of breath for a period of time, found that he was coughing up blood from his lungs. Instead of getting better, as he had hoped, the condition deteriorated quickly, until he could barely breathe. By the time his wife got him to the hospital, he had developed double pneumonia. Because of his serious health condition and exhaustion, exacerbated by his chronic coughing, he was put on drugs to alleviate the symptoms. In spite of the doctors' best efforts and the use of antibiotics and intravenous feeding, the lung refused to heal. After about a month, x-rays were taken and Richard Mott was told that he had a malignant tumor in his right lung. Unless this lung was surgically removed, he was warned, he would not have more than "three months to live."

It was, according to Mr. Mott, hard to imagine the state of shock he was in. He was asked to sign a paper giving the doctors permission to remove his lung. It was also explained to him that there were five or six malignant areas, and that the situation would get progressively worse. With the lung removed, the doctors estimated that he would be able to stretch the three months allotted to him to a year.

When his wife and daughter heard the bad news, they urged him to leave the hospital and try some form of alternative treatment that might offer a chance to regain his health. Mrs. Mott was a vegetarian who had done a great deal of reading in the area of natural medicine. She felt that turning in this direction was preferable to living out a year or so of his life under miserable circumstances. Though Mr. Mott had never shared his wife's interest in natural health practices, he now knew that conventional medicine had failed to help him and that he had nothing to look forward to except death.

A few days later he received an excited call from his wife that their daughter had contacted John Tobe, author and publisher of a health magazine, and that Mr. Tobe had recommended the well-known Dr. Max Warmbrand of Stamford, Connecticut. Dr. Warmbrand, after hearing Mr. Mott's story, had agreed to see him for a consultation. Meanwhile, Richard's doctors and nurses—even the chaplain—were doing their best to convince him to have his lung surgically removed. Instead, encouraged by his wife and daughter, Richard insisted on checking out of the hospital. When he left the next day, he was so exhausted by his illness that he was barely able to walk. The day after he came home, his wife drove him to see Dr. Warmbrand.

After giving Mr. Mott a thorough examination, Dr. Warmbrand noted that Mr. Mott was in an extreme state of weakness and nutritional imbalance as a consequence of a lifetime of poor dietary habits. This had included not only a constant fare of unwholesome foods, but also a chronic overuse of wine and hard liquor. "You must realize," Dr. Warmbrand said, "that in order to recover, you will have to begin rebuilding your body from scratch. Are you prepared," he asked, "to change every aspect of your living and eating pattern, so that you can give your body a chance to heal itself? Your body has a wonderful self-repair mechanism, but it can get better only if you make up your mind to eat to live rather than live to eat. If you sincerely agree to follow my advice—and not backslide—I will agree to accept you as a patient and try to help you."

At the time of his first visit to Dr. Warmbrand, Richard weighed more than 250 pounds. He was a voracious meat-eater, who would consume three or four steaks a week, meatballs, fowl and other flesh foods on weekdays, and a huge amount of roast beef on Sundays. The rest of his diet was made of coffee, tea, doughnuts, pastries, candy, white bread, refined flours and other dead foods. In addition, he would drink a pint of brandy and a six-pack of beer every day, and an additional fifth or two of hard liquor over the weekend.

After hearing this story, Dr. Warmbrand explained that his therapeutic approach consisted of rebuilding the body with all of the essential nutrients—particularly enzymes—through a proper nutritional regime. As one gets older and continues to deprive the system of enzymes because of poor eating habits, he pointed out, the body wastes pile up and eventually can contribute to the development of cancer. His practice was to put patients on a diet which supplied sufficient enzymes to metabolize food, and other vital elements which were needed to reverse the cancerous condition.

From this time on, there would be no more meats, bread, cakes, sugar, tea, coffee, chemicalized foods or alcohol in his diet. Mr. Mott heard Dr. Warmbrand's instructions with a sinking heart. As one whose meat-and-potatoes diet had been a daily necessity, he wondered whether this deprivation was worth the effort of saving his life. But then he thought, "Since my doctors give me only three months to live, why not give it a try?"

"You've eliminated just about everything that's worthwhile eating," Mott told the doctor, half in jest. "What can I eat instead?" The doctor's answer was: "What does a steer, a horse or a cow eat? Nothing but hay and grain, yet they grow to be big and healthy. And how many cancer operations do you hear performed on these animals?" He then told Mr. Mott that his new diet would mainly consist of raw fruits and vegetables of every variety, with grains, nuts, avocados and proteins. He emphasized the particular importance of "a green drink, combining the juices of lettuce, celery, carrot tops, beet-tops and other greens available in season."

A typical day's menu might consist of fruit, almonds and a large carrot juice, or else whole grains soaked overnight for breakfast; a big salad of a variety of raw vegetables with a little honey and juice for lunch; and another huge salad with a baked potato and avocado for dinner. Raw foods are more suitable for a cancer diet, Dr. Warmbrand explained, because the heat of cooking destroys the enzymes and alters the minerals and vitamins. The doctor also asked him to include garlic and cayenne pepper in his daily diet, and to throw out all of the drugs that had been given to him for a heart condition.

As far as the rest of the rebuilding regime, Dr. Warmbrand instructed Richard to get sufficient rest and sleep, and to take hot nightly baths with Epsom salts to open the pores of his skin so that the poisons could be drawn from his system. He gave him a number of simple but effective exercises to tone up his muscles to the degree that he was able to, given his extremely weakened physical condition. And finally, the doctor stressed the importance of thinking positively—and eliminating all morbid thoughts from his mind. Mrs. Mott listened carefully to Dr. Warmbrand's advice, since it would be largely up to her to prepare the food and see to it that her husband followed the regime.

Richard Mott was in such poor shape that at first he could barely get out of bed. His wife carefully prepared and served his food, and kept after him to see that he did not deviate from the nutritional program. To add even more precious nutrients to his system, she fed him sprouts and the juice of homegrown wheatgrass.

At first, Mr. Mott's diet seemed bland and tasteless; after a while, however, he began to look forward to the daily salads and other delicious raw foods which were awakening taste buds deadened by his former eating patterns. Within two months of following this diet faithfully, he began to feel considerably better. Meanwhile, even while in bed, he did whatever exercises he could, running his fingers up and down the wall, and raising and lowering his arms.

This went on for several months, until he reached the point where he could get up from bed and go to the bathroom alone. Every week Dr. Warmbrand examined him, checked on his progress with the nutritional program, and gave him chiropractic adjustments. Slowly, his strength began to return, and his eyes, which had been dull and yellowish, returned to their normal white.

Six months after he had gone on Dr. Warmbrand's regime, he was up and around the house, doing mild exercises and taking long walks in the countryside. Friends who had previously told each other that he was "like a walking dead man" now remarked on how well he looked. They could not believe that this was the same individual whose obituary they expected to appear any day in the local newspaper. Within this short period of time, his weight had gone down to 175 pounds, his heart showed considerable improvement and his lungs seemed perfectly normal.

A few months later he had to check out a foot injury that he had suffered many years ago when he was an athlete. He entered the same hospital where the doctors had advised a lung operation. When the doctors looked at his records, they were amazed to find that he was the former patient with lung cancer who had insisted on being discharged from the hospital without surgery.

With Mr. Mott's permission, they took x-rays of his lungs and compared these with previous x-rays that had shown tumorous masses in the right lung. They informed him that his lungs were now entirely clear and showed no evidence of cancer. Sputum samples were also negative. He had, according to the doctors, achieved 100% remission of the cancer.

When the doctors inquired about Mott's form of treatment, he explained that he had been on a natural nutritional regime consisting of eight ounces of juice twice a day, and vitamin supplements, just as Dr. Warmbrand had prescribed. He tried to relate, as clearly as he could, the healing concept behind this regime. They listened with great interest, but did not comment on what had happened.

Mr. Mott, who at the time of his original diagnosis was 75 years of age, remained faithfully on the program devised by Dr. Warmbrand for many years. He had the advantage of a cooperative and knowledgeable wife, who realized, as he did, that there was no going back to his former diet or way of living that was largely responsible for his illness. He took long daily hikes, tended a small garden that grew the organic vegetables he ate, slept well, and found time for rest and relaxation. To the best of his ability, he maintained a sense of personal calm and spiritual purpose which helped him handle the stress that is an inevitable part of everyone's life. Richard Mott survived for over ten years following the doctors' original bleak prognosis.

"A New Road to Recovery"

Hy Radin

In 1968 Hy Radin—in his late 50s—collapsed while walking in the street. He was taken to a hospital and diagnosed as having cancer of the spine. When he heard the dread word "cancer," he felt the overpowering shock which in his own words, "only cancer victims can understand." He was then told by his doctors that it was imperative for him to submit to surgery, otherwise nothing could be done to prolong his life much longer.

After a series of other diagnostic tests, including biopsies and scans, it was determined that the cancer had metastasized to the liver. Following the traditional method of treating this form of cancer, Hy Radin was given cobalt radiation. He was also put on an estrogen regime in the hope that this drug would reduce the enlarged prostate and nodules in that area. The treatment not only failed to reduce the swelling, but instead enlarged Mr. Radin's breasts. (For more than a year after taking the estrogen, he was impotent.)

While Hy was in the hospital, his wife had been trying to get the doctors to tell her the truth about her husband—to no avail. Finally the head nurse gave her the devastating news that he had only a short time to live. When Mr. Radin discovered that he was apparently so close to death, with no prospect of getting well, he decided to listen to the urging of his best friend, Lou Kashins. His response to the question by Lou, "What have you got to lose?" was to leave the hospital.

In a way, Hy Radin considered it his good fortune that the truth about his condition had not been kept from him. Otherwise, he may not have taken the path he did. Back at home, he had an opportunity to think things through and to make a free choice on what alternatives were open to him as a means of regaining his health—despite what he knew about the inevitability of his death. Looking back at the pattern of his lifestyle, he realized that he had been violating the rules of good health for many years, and that this had opened the way to his present cancerous condition.

As a young, successful businessman, he had habitually eaten extremely poor food, drank a good deal with his clients and smoked incessantly. When he was in his thirties, the first urgent signs of nutritional deficiency appeared in the form of diabetes. He went to a specialist in the field and was given the drug, Orinase, which he took for more than thirteen years.

The next indication of a serious dysfunction came in the form of arthritis. Once again, he engaged a top-flight physician in an effort to alleviate the painful ailment. This time he was treated unsuccessfully with an antiarthritic medication for more than three years. Meanwhile, his back had been giving him a great deal of trouble. As an ardent golfer, he sought the help of a specialist in bone problems, so that he could continue his favorite pastime. The diagnosis he received was that he was suffering from torn muscles in the lower part of his back. The treatment consisted of shortwave diathermy on the back, twice a week, for about six months.

With this record of chronic ailments in his background, Hy Radin realized that orthodox cancer therapies were not going to be of any help in restoring his health, and that he would have to consider a whole new direction if he was to get well. Meanwhile, he was fitted with a special metal brace, to prevent his spine from collapsing once again. It was at this point that he was ready to accept the advice of Lou Kashins, who had been interested in alternative health concepts for many years. In the past Hy had labelled his friend a faddist because of his belief in the importance of excellent nutrition. Now, however, he was more receptive to these ideas. He soon learned that Lou had a broad knowledge of nutrition and owned a large library of books relating to the subject of natural health. Following his friend's advice, Mr. Radin read *Superior Health Through Nutrition* and *How to Always Be Well*, both written by William Howard Hay. The information he read in this book was later to become the basis of the program which was so instrumental in restoring his health. Another book that proved helpful to him was *Food Is Your Best Medicine* by Henry Bieler, M.D.

With the knowledge he obtained in these books, and the help of his friend and others experienced in the biological approach to health, Hy Radin gradually changed his diet for the better and began to improve his condition. Eight weeks later—exactly twice the maximum time he had been given to survive—he was not only alive, but feeling somewhat stronger.

Although he was on this new recovery program, he was still taking estrogen and other drugs. Visiting a doctor for a routine examination, Hy Radin informed him that his condition was somewhat better and he described to the doctor the natural program he was following. After the doctor expressed skepticism about this form of natural therapy, Mr. Radin left, never again to return.

During the initial phase of his health program, Mr. Radin gave up the unwholesome foods he had been eating all of his adult life. Though he never became a vegetarian, he stopped eating meat, chicken and fowl, restricting himself to a small portion of fish daily. From that time on, fish and an occasional soft boiled egg were the only proteins he ate. Not more than 20% of his total intake was flesh protein. The bulk of his diet consisted of fresh vegetables and fruits, and all of the varieties of healthful foods he could purchase, preferably raw. Processed foods, particularly coffee, were no longer part of his diet.

Throughout the healing process, Hy made certain to drink a mixture of organic vegetable juices, such as carrot, celery and beets, four or five times daily, since these juices serve as an excellent source for nutrients and as a means of maintaining the acid-alkaline balance of the body. He continued to drink carrot and celery juice daily for the rest of his life, up until his death in his late 80s from natural causes—27 years from the time of his diagnosis.

As part of Dr. Hay's health restoration regime, Hy took two-quart enemas three or four times daily in order to keep his colon constantly cleansed of toxins. This is part of the Hay method of detoxification. Periodically, he did a three-day laxative purge as outlined by Norman W. Walker in his original book, *Fresh Vegetable and Fruit Juices.* In the course of this detoxification procedure, he ran into the usual problems such as fever, headache, and nausea, which may occur when the toxins leave the storage areas (cells, tissues and glands) and are collected by the bloodstream on their way to elimination from the body. Although he had an extremely severe case of cancer, he was not frightened by these symptoms. He knew they were reactions to be expected during the detoxification process.

About three months into the program, he found a doctor in Manhattan who had a nutritional practice (which was rare at the time). Mr. Radin was grateful for the doctor's knowledge and understanding of a different healing direction. It gave Hy a sense of security to have professional guidance, which is so important to cancer patients and difficult to achieve.

Approximately a year from the time he had initiated his repair program, he began to make great strides in recovering his health. An astonishing thing had happened: the diseased bone in his spine had been replaced with healthy tissue. The only weak spot that remained was in his back where cobalt had been used. Firstly, he was able to give up his back brace. Then his wheel chair and walk with crutches. Finally, he progressed to a walker. When he no longer needed the walker, he resumed working at his own business, resumed his favorite form of daily exercise—golf—and carried on his life activities normally. The diabetic and arthritic condition improved along with the cancer. Bone spurs on both heels disappeared, as did the aches and pains associated with his illness. Under no circumstances did he ever again take drugs.

Raw natural foods, for the most part, continued to be the major part of his diet. He also took supplements when they were needed. Summing up his own recovery and maintenance of health all those years, Hy Radin observed: "I have found from my own experience, and from other cases, that many individuals on this kind of program can do exceedingly well. Just stop what is causing the problem, and give Nature half a chance."

"My Body and My Life"

Lou Dina

In 1978 (in his late 20s) Lou Dina was diagnosed with a malignant form of lymphoma. His case history, however, really began many years before when, as a child, he suffered from constant throat problems. His poor resistance made him prone to strep throat, tonsillitis, colds and flu. Like most children he received the standard inoculations and ate the standard 1950s American "balanced" diet which included lots of dairy, fats, sugars, soft drinks and junk food.

In response to his frequent throat infections, Lou's tonsils were removed in the 4th grade. In the 5th grade he began to have a severe problem with his right elbow joint. It would swell and become quite painful at irregular intervals. The problem would go on for a few weeks and then disappear mysteriously. As time went on, the frequency, duration, and intensity increased to the point where something had to be done. An orthopedic surgeon found that x-rays indicated a cyst was affecting the bone inside the elbow joint. The doctor scraped out the joint. Bone was grafted from the right hip to fill the hole eaten out by the cyst. There was no diagnosis of malignancy and the problem seemed to go away after surgery.

But Lou's diet remained the same as did his general weak state of health and he continued to suffer a high incidence of colds, sore throats and flu. In 1975 he began to have a swelling and soreness in his left wrist, similar to the elbow problem in the 5th grade. Even wrapped in an ace bandage, the slightest wrist movement caused intense pain. At first, the problem surfaced every 4 months or so and lasted a few weeks. A doctor diagnosed gout, but the prescribed "cure" proved ineffectual. Finally, in 1978 another doctor took one look at the severely distended wrist (now the size of a tennis ball) and insisted Lou check into a hospital immediately. A biopsy revealed a malignant form of lymphoma in the bones and lymph system. A second biopsy indicated that Lou had lymphoma in the lymph node in his left armpit.

A whole battery of tests followed, including a CT scan and various other imaging diagnostic devices. As Lou puts it, "I had taken so many radioactive isotopes that I was able to spin the needle on a 'Geiger counter' located in the nuclear medicine waiting room. I was a pretty hot number!"

At this point the left wrist bone, almost totally consumed by the cancer, was the consistency of soft mush. He couldn't move it at all. A series of radiation treatments to the wrist and arm reduced the mass so that it looked more normal, but the wrist remained sore and weak. The radiation burned all the hair from his arm and caused the skin to dry and crack. This was followed by one chemotherapy treatment which produced a three-day migraine headache and nausea. Lou was given codeine for pain relief for his head and wrist. Despite his numerous questions about the treatment and its side effects, doctors gave him minimal feedback or explanations.

Lou was hungry for understanding of his condition and so began his own search for answers. He consumed any available books on the subject, networked with recovered patients, contacted clinics, obtained literature from FACT and attended an annual FACT Cancer/Nutrition Convention in Detroit. Immediately following that convention, he decided to suspend all conventional treatment until he had explored the alternatives further. He admits that at the time he was simultaneously encouraged and petrified by his discoveries. As an engineer, he had been trained to methodically investigate and seek out the root cause(s). The alternatives, therefore, made tremendous sense to him, but at the same time, he was scared of deviating from the advice of the orthodox medical professionals, who, after all, had the imprimatur of years of the most "advanced" scientific and medical training. Despite the fact that he found himself caught in a severe emotional quandary as he gathered all the information he could, Lou made the conscious decision to take charge of his treatment: "It was **my** body and **my** life. No longer would I relinquish these decisions to others and blindly follow."

Lou wrote out a three-page list of questions and made an appointment with his oncologist. Insisting on clear answers to his many questions, he gave the doctor a 90-minute exam. The doctor was accommodating, but by the end of the interview, his patient was leaning strongly toward alternative treatments. When Lou told him this, the doctor became very defensive and upset, relating examples of three or four close relatives who had died of cancer and how he had done everything to save them. The oncologist claimed his track record was above average and told Lou that he considered these "so-called alternatives" quackery.

The doctor's responses had helped Lou decide in favor of alternative treatment. Two years after leaving orthodox care and adhering to a metabolic therapy, Lou was offered a promotion by his company on the condition that he obtain a clean bill of health from his original oncologist. After a thorough examination, this same oncologist declared Lou totally free of cancer. "What amazed me," Lou noted at the time, "was that he never once expressed any curiosity as to how I had done it. Amazing!"

Initially, Lou based his metabolic program on the Kelley plan, and followed it to the letter. He consulted Dr. Kelley totally via mail, with fluid samples, a massive questionnaire, and medical reports. After about 6 months Lou decided to attend the John Richardson Clinic in Berkeley, California. This program had many elements in common with Kelley's. In fact, Lou discovered that most of the successful alternatives he had become acquainted with shared many similarities that were integral to reestablish the integrity of the body and thereby rebuild the immune system. Among these, Lou delineated the following:

1. Whole, natural foods, largely in their raw, organic state, were used abundantly. This included vegetables, fruits, nuts, grains, etc. All additives, preservatives, refined sugar, white flour, adulterated meats, soft drinks and junk food were avoided.

2. The body needed cleansing inside and out to assist in the elimination of accumulated waste products and toxins. Various methods were used including high enemas, flushes and purges.

3. Liberal quantities of freshly-squeezed carrot juice were consumed. He typically drank a combination of carrot juice mixed with celery juice. He would often add other juices such as spinach or beet. This was an important part of the program.

4. Supplements were added to his diet to help correct specific individual deficiencies. He took pancreatic enzymes, liver supplements, bone supplements, and numerous others. These supplements must be tailored to the specific needs of each individual patient. The assistance of a knowledgeable professional, such as available from FACT, is indicated.

5. A "take charge attitude" helps reduce stress and improve well-being. These factors are shown to make a significant difference in a patient's ability to recuperate. Imagery, relaxation, and a positive outlook seem to assist the body in restoring normal functioning of the various glands and organs.

6. Exercise as appropriate for the condition of the patient is important. The goal is to get oxygen and blood pumping to nourish cells and assist in elimination. It is not appropriate for sick persons to wear themselves out. Moderation is in order.

7. He highly recommends the assistance of a professional health practitioner well-versed in biological alternatives. A tested and proven practitioner can keep you on the right track. (Lou felt that FACT was the best source for guidance).

8. Stay involved. Hippocrates said, "Physician, heal thyself." It is your body and your life.

To this Lou adds one more piece of the puzzle: "I am convinced that emotional problems and severe emotional trauma often play a significant role in causing cancer. I believe this was very true in my case. I have worked very hard to eliminate suppressed anger and resentment from my life. This is why I feel so strongly about people getting involved in their treatment. Somehow, when you become actively involved, attitudes change and this affects the body's chemical and electrical processes in a very positive manner."

To date Lou has not had any recurrence of cancer. His wrist bone has grown back completely and functions fairly normally, though it remains somewhat deformed and weak from the devastation wrought by cancer and radiation treatments. Since full recovery, he occasionally strays from his diet, reverting to foods and habits that are not conducive to health. When he doesn't feel well, or if the wrist hurts a lot (sometimes due to weather changes), he'll "clean up my act" and return to a healthier diet, following the steps outlined above. Having learned that his body has some inherent weaknesses, and that going back to the standard junk foods leads to problems, he admits that, undoubtedly, the best course is to stay on a healthy diet all the time.

He has also found that his health is impaired during periods of severe emotional stress, especially in conjunction with a poor diet. The best news is that he now has confidence that he has rebuilt his health, strengthened his defenses and immune system by going to the source rather than attacking symptoms. That, he feels, is the essence and the beauty of a good alternative treatment.

"Raw Diet Beats Cancer"

Louise Greenfield

In December of 1977 two hard lumps located close to each other were removed from Louise Greenfield's right breast. A biopsy indicated that she had "an infiltrating adeno-carcinoma of the breast." Her surgeon said she must have an operation within ten days. He recommended a modified mastectomy and implied how lucky she was that they no longer advised radical mastectomies.

Totally unprepared for this pronouncement, she was thrown into absolute terror. She did not smoke and had cut down drastically on beef and junk foods for ten years, innocently thinking these measures would save her from ever hearing this dreadful news.

She and her husband knew of Dr. Jack Goldstein, author of *Triumph Over Disease—by Fasting and Natural Diet*. In this book, which reads like an adventure story, Dr. Goldstein, a podiatrist and nutritional consultant in Livonia, Michigan, tells how he cured himself of a devastating case of ulcerative colitis.

Since Louise's mind had, in her own words, "stopped working," from the shock of her cancer diagnosis, she never even thought of Dr. Goldstein. But, fortunately, her husband suggested they seek his advice.

The doctor had her come in for a consultation and took her history. He said it was to her benefit that she had not had radiation or chemotherapy because it would result in the destruction of normal cells. He drew up a diet plan for her and, with his help, she was on her way to defeating her cancer.

It is now over 25 years later and without having had the mastectomy, radiation, chemotherapy or any drugs, Louise remains in good health. She functions normally, and has, as she proudly states, "two breasts."

The diet consisted of raw foods for the first two months. During that time, she was allowed nothing cooked and nothing hot, not even a cup of herb tea. It was basically a type of diet designed to make things easy for that important organ, the liver. It consisted mainly of raw vegetable juice followed by raw blended salad, whole salad without dressing, whole fruit, raw milk, unsalted cheese, raw unsalted nuts, and some seeds. The first thing she had to do was buy a juicer and a heavy-duty blender.

These foods were to be eaten slowly to allow digestion to start in the mouth. Nuts were to be chewed to a cream. Water for drinking and cooking was to be distilled. She was to avoid taking any medication and was to have nothing artificial in her food, and, of course, nothing cooked.

In the beginning most of the foods tasted awful. Only the threat of a mastectomy made her stick to it. She spent hours dreaming about hot food. She would have sold her soul for a hot vegetable!

Louise begged for hot tea at the very least. But Dr. Goldstein said the first four months—indeed the first year—were crucial in changing her internal chemistry. During the first two months on the raw diet, she gradually lost twenty pounds, going from a size twelve to a size eight. Her stools changed drastically. They became very light in color, also soft, enormous, and frequent. Indeed, she had found that, "a raw diet is a sure cure for constipation!"

After two months, Dr. Goldstein allowed Louise to use tahini dressing and eat a few lightly steamed vegetables. As Louise puts it, "I will never forget my first hot food—it was an utterly plain baked potato, no salt, no butter. But every bite was heavenly."

When nearly a year had gone by, Dr. Goldstein allowed her occasional fish and chicken. The first time she ate fish she became extremely uncomfortable from the unaccustomed load on her stomach.

It's important to mention that Louise had a physical condition that caused her many problems when she changed to the raw diet. Two years before the cancer diagnosis she had developed colitis—inflammation of the colon with attendant gas, pain and diarrhea. Her family doctor put her on a bland diet which relieved the pain but caused chronic constipation. When she began the new diet, you can imagine the difficulty her system had tolerating raw foods. The diet was very time-consuming to prepare and clean up afterward. Sometimes she felt like a rabbit.

However, she persisted because anything was better than losing a breast. After a few months on the raw regime, the colitis improved. It continued to improve except when she experienced unusual stress; as a rule she had neither diarrhea nor constipation and very little pain.

One reason she was so determined to maintain the diet was because she had two friends who had been stricken by cancer. Both accepted conventional medical treatment, submitting to countless operations, radiation and chemotherapy. Both developed unhealthy brown complexions and terrible fatigue. Both died.

On occasion when she was unduly stressed, hard painful lumps appeared in one of her breasts. At these times, she eliminated all cooked items, got more rest, and in three or four weeks the lumps disappeared. She called it, "a miracle—a miracle of my body."

I would like to note several differences in Louise's program from the usual metabolic therapy. For the first year, Louise was on a total vegetarian diet, totally raw in its beginning stages. This is not necessarily recommended by every practitioner for everyone. A total vegetarian diet is deficient for individuals who require flesh food for competent balance and healthy cell production. It should also be noted that Dr. Goldstein's system differs from most other practitioners of metabolic therapies in that it does not include, except for fasting, routine detoxification.

"Why Me?"

Betty Fowler

Betty Fowler, retired former director of the Fowler School of Practical Ballet in New York, was diagnosed as having skin cancer in 1971. She had previous indications of serious health problems and a number of upsetting experiences with conventional medicine. During a pregnancy, at the age of 23, she received x-ray treatments for a pilonidal cyst. Later, it had to be cut and drained for a period of more than two years, and finally was removed.

When she was 37, she had a partial hysterectomy, in the course of which a large tumor was removed. Two years later, a brown mole which had been on her cheek since the age of four began to enlarge and was surgically excised. A biopsy at the time indicated that it was nonmalignant. Then, at the age of forty, Betty had a small growth under her left breast removed. Once again, the diagnosis on the basis of a biopsy was nonmalignant.

In 1969, her gynecologist recommended that she take estrogen because of her partial hysterectomy. She took this drug for several months and stopped when white spots appeared on her thighs and a growth developed under the arch of her left foot. The doctor diagnosed the growth as being a tumor and surgically removed it. This too was then declared to be nonmalignant. At the same time, the skin specialist removed some small growths on her face, forehead and wrist.

The same year, Mrs. Fowler developed a chronic high temperature and was given antibiotics to bring down the fever. She began to suffer a number of distressing symptoms, including severe gas, inability to focus her eyes or to read, muscular weaknesses and cramps. The cramps were so painful that she would scream and awaken her whole family. Next, her hair turned gray and became brittle. On top of this, her face hurt to the point where the pain became intolerable. After suffering from this intense pain for nearly three years—from 1968 to 1971—and going from doctor to doctor in an effort to find relief—she was given a battery of tests and informed that the condition was merely psychosomatic.

When the pain became too excruciating to bear, Mrs. Fowler visited the surgeon who had previously removed several growths. A week later he told her that a growth on her face was cancerous. She was hospitalized, and subjected to further x-rays and other tests. Now a biopsy confirmed a malignancy and she was told that she might have to wait six months before the section that had been taken from her face would heal. Within a few months the pain became so constant and severe that she visited the surgeon and was now informed that the condition was not, as he had first thought, a simple basal epithelioma, *but that possibly it could be melanoma* and might have already metastasized into the mouth. Recalling her reaction at the time, she remembers thinking, "You have cancer." She felt it was a sentence of death by painful means. Her second thought was, "Why me?"

After a two-year period and unsuccessful surgical results, her surgeon suggested another modality. Special chemicals, she was told, would be applied to her face, and where an area was revealed to be cancerous, the specialist would remove it surgically. If the areas that were cut did not heal, it was explained to her, a good plastic surgeon could repair the damage.

For several reasons, Mrs. Fowler decided not to follow this path. First, the expense was beyond her means; and second, she did not wish to accept the possibility of a face more mutilated with scars than she already had from previous surgeries. There already existed a large lump between her lip and chin. The skin specialist insisted that she start the treatment immediately. Instead, Mrs. Fowler decided to cut off all communication with him and began to search for an alternative way to combat the cancer.

She had come across a book by Dr. Max Gerson and was very impressed by what she read. On making inquiries, she was disappointed to discover that he was deceased. Visiting a health food store, she found a book called *New Hope for Cancer Victims* by Dr. William Donald Kelley. In this book, Dr. Kelley described the symptoms of a cancer patient which virtually matched her own—flatulence, hot flashes, fatigue, bleeding gums, abdominal pains, muscular weakness and a change in the color of her hair.

When she revealed to the store owner that she had cancer and wanted to contact Dr. Kelley, Betty Fowler was advised to call FACT. Through FACT, Mrs. Fowler was given information and knowledge to help explain the biological approach to cancer. Like many other cancer patients, she remained in touch with FACT throughout her repair program to consult whenever she needed advice and to share in a sense of encouragement and support. In 1972 she visited Dr. Kelley and was given the Kelley test. He informed her that her form of cancer had been particularly painful because it had involved a nerve. In the course of examining and questioning her, he also found serious nutritional deficiencies.

All her life before this, she had abused her body with a fairly typical diet of coffee four or five times a day, hamburgers and french fries, and other junk foods. Routinely she would take aspirin for her severe migraines, and laxatives to relieve her constipation. Now, under Dr. Kelley's nutritional regime, she was placed on an entirely different nutritional program, including carrot juice, raw vegetables and fruits, nuts, grains, etc. The new diet also included a number of supplements to provide sorely-needed vitamins, minerals, enzymes, glandulars and other nutrients. In addition, Mrs. Fowler was placed on a regimen of enemas; this continued for a whole year. Even while on this program, she continued to hope for some medical miracle—a drug, injection or treatment—that would in itself make the cancer disappear.

At first, as is so often the case when an individual begins a biorepair program, her body had strange reactions to changes stimulated by the improved nutritional material. Among these symptoms were stomach aches, gas, nausea, muscular weakness, depression, a slight fever and other flu-like reactions. Dr. Kelley explained to her that she was dislodging a lifetime of poisons which were now trying to find their way out of her body. The flare-ups and other distresses were a typical part of the healing process.

In time, every area where she had been previously operated upon began to erupt with large boils. They would recede when she detoxified with enemas and/or colonics and come back as she went through her eliminative process stimulated by the metabolic program. During this period she also had offensive breath and a coated and ridged tongue. One morning she woke to discover that the "blue blob" on her chin had broken open and was leaking a very thick, sticky pus. The lump drained intermittently until, some months later, it finally healed.

Around this time she visited her family physician, who examined the "blue blob" and informed her that it did not appear to be cancerous. He suggested instead that it was probably a sebaceous cyst. She told him that *three separate biopsies had diagnosed it as being malignant.*

The following year a much improved Mrs. Fowler visited Dr. Kelley for a retest. She asked him if it was safe to have the lump on her chin surgically removed. When he answered in the affirmative, she visited a specialist in New York City for the surgical procedure. The doctor diagnosed the area as the largest mucous cyst he had ever seen. It took three visits to remove a cyst of that size. When the procedure was over, the surgeon gave Mrs. Fowler a note certifying that the cyst he had removed from her chin was not cancerous. This was her proof that her metabolic program had indeed worked.

In the twenty-five-plus years since then, Mrs. Fowler has adhered to the biological principles of good health as outlined by Dr. Kelley. She has had herself retested periodically, and is healthy. She now lives in a rural area in Washington. In this natural and relaxed setting, she works full time, feels physically and emotionally fit and looks forward to a long, productive life.

"God Will Show Me the Way"

Doris Sokosh

Doris is a lively woman in her early 70s who first noted soreness and discomfort in her right breast late in 1970. She was a "houseworker" at the time and had "worked hard all my life." The breast appeared bruised. Shortly before that time, she had developed a discharge from the navel and an unusual vaginal discharge. She said that her periods were also "not right" (they were "dark and light"), and she knew she had a cyst "down below." She went to her chiropractor who suggested a medical checkup.

Following the medical examination, she underwent a radical mastectomy on October 31, 1971. Ten days later, a hysterectomy was performed "to prevent further spread." The procedures were done at Norwalk Hospital in Connecticut. The attending physician was Dr. Abrams. She was then referred to Dr. DeCorato for postoperative follow-up and care.

Over the course of the next one and a half years, five skin grafts were done to cover the operative site, using skin from the thigh. She also had a "small amount" of radiation. During this period there was a lot of bleeding and drainage from the chest, a great deal of pain ("like a knife") and the graft areas on her legs would not heal. She was given drugs for "pain, depression and stress." Her weight kept dropping and reached as low as 75 pounds. She was referred to Dr. Corso who ordered a GI x-ray series. She said he "gave no answers" but told her family she was in "bad shape." By October 1974, she was no longer able to care for herself and moved to her mother's home. At that point she became quite weak and was bedridden. In addition, her mind was so foggy that she was unable to recognize people she knew.

Doris' husband came to the FACT office from Connecticut. Doris was on pain medication after six surgical procedures and was scheduled for a seventh. Her case was far advanced.

I suggested that they consider a clinic, but she was unable to be moved and even too weak to make visits to a doctor's office. I was left with no choice but to provide the guidance she desperately needed. Her husband and I talked at length and he left with some books to help him understand a different concept of treatment in order to help Doris.

He was advised to start her on juices, mainly carrot. Also, she was to drink only distilled water and begin daily enemas. Her desire for food and her ability to digest it was very limited, but whatever she was able to ingest was of the highest quality for maximum benefit. Steamed vegetables were added to the diet next, and two months later she was started on fish one day a week. Also, it was recommended that she take enzymes, Greenlife (a high-quality chlorophyll product that acts as a potent multivitamin) and glandulars (including thymus for immunity and liver).

During the course of the next four months, she experienced many healing "reactions": fevers, breaking out in hives "all over the body," chest drainage, hemorrhoids, legs becoming very cold (for which she applied heated castor oil packs) and severe insomnia for about two weeks.

By February of 1975, she had progressed to the point where she was able to dress herself and had started to walk. She was gaining about one pound per week. By March she weighed 117 pounds and was able to return to her home with the help of members of her congregation.

Under FACT's guidance, she was now eating steamed vegetables, salads, baked potatoes, eggs every other day and, occasionally, chicken breasts. Daily enemas were continued. One year after the initial contact with FACT, she began receiving regular massages and colonics three times per week from a professional therapist. At a year and a half, she began to feel "really good."

Mrs. Sokosh feels that her recovery had a great deal to do with the support that she received. Her husband was "with me every minute." She received great "love, support and prayer from my congregation" which gave her confidence; and "the powerful support and guidance from Ruth Sackman and FACT were vital to my complete recovery."

I would also attribute her recovery to her faith. Soon after she contacted me, she said "If God wants to take me in his arms, I am ready to go. If he doesn't, he will show me the way." This peacefulness with her condition gave her body the opportunity to function without stress. It released the natural ability for self-healing to take effect.

Doris has written a book, *Triumph Over Cancer, Recipes for Recovery*. The book has a more detailed description of her case history and recipes she created for her recovery.

(This case history was compiled with the help of Herman Lerner, MD, 2001.)

Summation

In reviewing these and other case histories of former cancer patients, I think I can safely conclude that certain common factors exist, even though the form of cancer and personal circumstances obviously differed from individual to individual.

First, all the patients who regained their health, when faced with the reality that they could not survive long with orthodox treatments, chose alternative pathways to recovery. Second, most of these cancer patients were fortunate in being able to find competent practitioners who matched the repair program to the individual, not the individual to the program. Third, the biological repair regimes in each instance included as major factors: improved nutritional regimes, metabolic competence, immune enhancement and a program of thorough detoxification of body wastes.

At the same time, the repair programs did not ignore other essential aspects of the whole-body approach, such as exercise, sufficient sleep and rest, and avoidance, to the degree that was feasible, of stress and emotional turmoil. Usually, the cancer patients were assisted throughout their program by family members or friends who were sympathetic to the biological approach and cooperative in ensuring that it was carried out effectively. They avoided a negative atmosphere.

Finally, in each instance, there were *common traits* which seem to be essential for the restoration of health in all cancer patients. These important traits include a *strong will* to survive whatever the obstacles that arise, a *belief that the body* is capable of restoring health, taking responsibility for decisions and a feeling that *life has an intrinsic value* which makes existence itself worth fighting for.

Appendix II:
Questions and Answers

The nearer a person is to the truth,
the more intelligent and simple they are.
—ANTON CHEKHOV, PHYSICIAN AND PLAYWRIGHT

In the course of my activities at FACT, I have been asked thousands of questions relating not only to the biological treatment of cancer, but to other aspects of health and disease. Sometimes the questions come as a result of people phoning or writing for information, or at question-and-answer periods at conferences, seminars or radio and television appearances.

I find it very significant that the same kinds of questions keep coming up constantly—even among people who are close to FACT—despite the fact that the information has appeared in *Cancer Forum* or other material that we publish. It is my feeling that this indicates either I have not been able to explain FACT's views clearly enough or else people who are seeking information from FACT are conditioned to using a different concept of healing. We are accustomed to using prescribed drugs that focus on alleviating symptoms instead of seeking causes and taking the considerable time it takes to repair the breakdown. It may be this kind of orientation that is hampering the public's receptivity to a different approach.

I have included a number of questions which provide an opportunity to deal with areas where there exists a considerable amount of contradictory, unproven, controversial or even erroneous information. Hopefully, the material in this chapter will serve as a guide to correct the flood of misinformation which is, unfortunately, so widely disseminated. The questions and answers are arranged, as much as possible, under appropriate categories, so that the material is more readily accessible to the reader.

The Biological Repair Concept

Q. *I've read somewhere that no repair system can actually cure cancer, only correct its causes. Is this so?*

A. It is absolutely true that one must correct causes. If that keeps the patients healthy and cancer-free for the rest of their life, that should be considered a cancer cure. If you can make the biological repair, you can indeed restore an individual to good health. If I don't use the term "cure," it's because I would rather label the problem a biological breakdown instead of cancer, and what you do is repair the breakdown, thereby, restoring the patient to health. In this way I feel that the healing process is more accurately described and the results are long-lasting.

Q. *How do you judge when a patient has had a successful biological repair?*

A. I can't quite specify the period of time that has to elapse before someone can be said to have recovered. Each person undertakes healing with their own strengths and weaknesses which determines the time it takes to complete the repair. Most of the clinics and clinicians using biorepair feel that a program should be adhered to for at least 2 years. I hope people will avoid ever returning to the lifestyle originally responsible for the breakdown.

Q. *How do you know when an individual is so ill that no repair system can possibly save his or her life?*

A. There is no accurate yardstick for measuring whether or not a person is beyond recovery. When a patient has had too much radiation or chemotherapy to the point where there is severe damage to a vital process, such as, liver function, immune function, kidney function, or a dysfunction of any other system, it's more difficult for them to reverse the damage successfully. This is especially true because of the very aggressive forms of chemotherapy in use today. There are certain aspects of a patient who has had radiation or chemotherapy which provide clues as to why it might be difficult for them to recover. They may, for example, begin to build up fluids in the lungs or peritoneal area. This does not mean that it is impossible to treat such a patient successfully, but it is an extremely difficult condition to overcome. Another serious handicap occurs when the patient has had a surgical procedure which alters the normal biological processes. This does not refer to cases where one kidney is removed, since it is possible for an individual to function with only one kidney. When bypasses are done, however, it might interfere with normal function of the body; therefore, making the full repair difficult.

Q. *Would you recommend that an individual go on a biological repair program under any circumstances?*

A. Yes, but cautiously. If a patient has had an enormous amount of chemotherapy, detoxification should be undertaken before any metabolic program is started. Supervision is important under most circumstances, but even more so when patients have been subjected to toxic therapies. Otherwise, the nutritional and other biological changes provoked by the repair program could bring about troublesome and unpredictable reactions (flare-ups) which require experienced guidance. The toxic chemicals which may have been stored in the cells or lymphatics as a result of chemotherapy may be released into the bloodstream without the control used when it was administered. This toxicity in the bloodstream causes the patient to have symptoms of toxemia.

Q. *Why do you object to the term "holistic?"*

A. I don't object to it; I just prefer the word "wholistic." The people who bandy the term about, don't, for the most part, have enough in-depth understanding of what taking care of the whole human system entails. Taking care of the whole body is a complex process which goes far beyond, for example, just changing a person's nutritional pattern, detoxifying, doing some spinal manipulation or psychological counselling. Yet many people who are doing nutritional therapy are naive and rarely understand the complications involved in a truly wholistic system of repair. I know a doctor, for instance, who even uses chemotherapy, plus some of the so-called botanical drugs, and he calls himself a "holistic healer." Others who utilize radiation will still insist that their approach is "holistic" if they include a proper diet. The way I prefer to use the term is that the individual must be on a *biologically safe and comprehensive system of repair.*

The Conventional Approach

Q. *Would you ever suggest conventional treatments such as chemotherapy or radiation for someone who has cancer?*

A. Yes, I have, but under special circumstances. I would like to see a biorepair system instituted immediately after surgery as a routine protocol instead of chemotherapy or radiation. I would like to see this done before harming the patient irreparably. If the patient is not responding because of an irreparable breakdown in body chemistry, and biological therapies have been unable to help then, of course, the patient should consider conventional treatment to achieve tumor reduction to buy time. The same thing pertains to individuals who are simply not competent or caring enough to adhere to a biorepair program properly.

In this vein, I want to speak of one patient to whom I suggested chemotherapy. This woman had been a participant in FACT for many years. She attended all of the health lectures possible, was interested in everything that was going on in health circles, and read everything she could in the area of biorepair. Then, one day, she developed a tumor in the breast; this was probably due to misinterpreting the information she had received, not understanding the physiological process of healing, and using the information without enough experience or good judgement.

Thinking she was now an authority in natural healing, she proceeded simultaneously to subject herself to every kind of therapy she had learned about, not understanding that you can overstimulate the body's healing mechanism. When the immune system is overstimulated, the toxins are released more rapidly than the eliminatory organs can process the toxic overload. As a result, this woman was getting sicker and more exhausted every day, and there was nothing one could tell her that would make her back off. She was not even applying much-needed detoxification techniques competently. Her liver began to swell and she could hardly lift herself from the bed.

I then suggested that she start a system of mild chemotherapy to depress the immune mechanism slightly because it was *overstimulated*. Of course, she refused to do this, since it appeared to her that my advice went counter to her healing orientation. She then became frightened and looked for professional guidance. She selected a center specializing in immunotherapy—*the worst choice she could possibly make at that particular time. It was physiologically contraindicated.* (A good system improperly applied is hazardous.) She stimulated an already overstimulated immune system. A few days after undergoing the treatment at the clinic she died. She had no understanding of the physiological process in using a biorepair program. This woman failed to heal herself; there are people who undertake healing others with the same limited understanding.

Q. *How do you explain the resistance of so many conventional doctors to nutritional therapy?*

A. In the first place, they haven't received the proper training in nutrition at their medical schools. Nutrition is to the human body what gasoline is to a car; the body cannot function without proper fuel. The nutritional approach, within the framework of biorepair, just isn't part of their orientation. But I also have to qualify the question, because it assumes that orthodox medicine is, per se, against nutrition. Three decades ago, when we started FACT, we got feedback from patients of their doctors' hostility to the nutritional concept of repair. Some of the oncologists absolutely forbade patients on chemotherapy from getting involved in an improved nutritional program. That situation was commonplace. Today it is far different. The acceptance of nutrition has developed to the point where the American Cancer Society has held seminars on nutrition; where some of the major medical institutions have nutritional counselors on their staffs; and where the National Cancer Institute is offering a nutritional brochure on cancer and nutrition (available by calling 1-800-4-CANCER). More and more, conventional research is validating the important role of diet in health and disease.

Q. *Would you say that there has been greater acceptance of the biological approach to cancer on the part of the medical profession?*

A. Definitely. We feel that the climate today is much more favorable regarding the biological viewpoint than it was even a short time ago. We are beginning to find that the information coming to us from conventional sources is more in harmony with what we have been disseminating for years. There is beginning to be a greater meeting of the minds, and not only in the area of nutrition.

Just a few years ago I was in a debate with a doctor—as a matter of fact, an oncological surgeon, who was representing the American Cancer Society—who presented a point of view on cancer that was very much like ours. In addition to nutrition, she spoke about such cancer-inducing factors as stress, drugs and other toxic materials. She pointed out that people don't want to change their lifestyles; instead, they are looking for short-cuts, easy ways out, so that they can eat all the bad food to which they are accustomed and then take a pill to overcome the harm. Of course, I was in total agreement with her. To grow we all have to start at some point to reach the optimum pathway to understanding.

Q. *I read an article recently in which it was claimed that there was a steady increase in the cancer survival time. Do you agree?*

A. I think we can agree, in some instances, that conventional treatments have extended the survival time. Not necessarily because the treatments in themselves are creating the extension, but because better diagnostic techniques are finding the tumors earlier than in the past. As a result, the increased survival time comes from starting the clock earlier, not necessarily from an improvement in cancer management. There are also some instances where time has been added.

In other words, we are suggesting that the *survival statistics* are showing a rise primarily because of earlier detection, not because they are accomplishing much more by starting treatment earlier. Sometimes, in fact, the earlier detection of a tumor can place the patient in "a treatment syndrome," and these days, this syndrome is something to question, especially if it is a mistaken diagnosis. Unfortunately, techniques today are becoming more aggressive, and the evaluation as to whether a particular treatment has been beneficial will have to be measured in the future. Time has to be a component in determining success or failure of a system or therapy related to cancer.

Too often, routine chemotherapy has been known to cause complications and possibly death so that patients unfortunately can die from the treatment rather than the cancer.

So, too, routine x-ray may put the patient at risk. On the basis of the facts, you should participate in making the choice instead of expecting the doctor to routinely decide what is to be done next. Even the insurance companies caution against unnecessary x-rays. It's up to you to assume some responsibility and to collect as much data as you can and then evaluate what's best, and make your own informed decision. Patients should be aware that doctors prescribe by offering accepted protocols or they risk malpractice suits or their professional license.

I'm sure someone is going to slap my wrist for this next statement. The American Cancer Society advocates early detection as a primary factor in effecting a cancer cure. And yet, as I have tried to show, all that early detection does at best is to improve the statistics. In uterine cancer the survival time has actually decreased, perhaps because of too aggressive treatment modalities. Perhaps some of these patients could have gone on living if they had not been subjected to such aggressive therapies. For example, an article that appeared in the *New England Journal of Medicine* showed that radiation after surgery has shortened the lives of some lung cancer patients.

I had an occasion to be on a panel discussion with a doctor who told me about a particular patient who was enjoying a 28-year survival period without any treatment. The doctor told me that this can sometimes happen with melanoma. I had heard this before and couldn't argue, but what I did say to her was, "if you had chosen one of the conventional treatments, if you had given her radiation and/or chemotherapy, the treatments might have precluded the opportunity to survive." This oncologist couldn't help but nod her head. So once again I suggest that every individual who is in a situation where a choice has to be made as to the best type of treatment should learn all the basic facts, and decide in partnership with their doctor which direction to take. This relieves the doctor of full responsibility.

Q. *Do you think that surgery in breast cancer is indicated in any circumstance?*

A. There are instances where surgery has merit. Sometimes, relieving the tumor load means that the body does not have to break it down on its own and get rid of it through other processes, and this can be less burdensome for the repair process. There are individuals who should be relieved of a tumor, because it will cause too much mental stress, which interferes with recovery. Cancer patients often feel the tumor as a palpable presence, and are constantly anxious that it might be growing. This kind of individual should definitely have the tumor removed if it is at all feasible. After this, they can follow a biorepair process. In any situation where the patient's personality will lead to a state of depression or panic, and not allow them to relax and make the proper decisions, the tumor should definitely be surgically removed, providing the removal itself does not hamper the body's ability to make the biorepair later on.

Q. *Should the question of removing a tumor be left up to the doctor?*

A. No. You should not leave decisions entirely with someone else. Feeling in control and taking responsibility for your health with the doctor's cooperation is wiser. As a matter of fact, research has shown that the patient who feels in control does better than the person who feels helpless. As difficult as it may seem, it may be necessary for patients to become completely informed and, in consultation with their doctors, make the final decision. There are some surgical procedures, especially bypasses, which preclude the body's ability to make a biorepair.

I think I ought to spell out some of the problems involved here, because it is very easy to misinterpret what I am saying. For instance, some doctors remove large segments of the colon even though the tumor is small. This means that much of the natural colon activity is lost. Bypasses are sometimes done to give patients relief of symptoms. This deprives a segment of the body of adequate blood supply needed to carry nourishment to that area. It is a tremendous handicap to the repair process. In much the same way, bypasses of the pancreas will prevent all of the pancreatic enzymes from performing their digestive role.

Q. *In the last few decades, hundreds of millions of dollars have been poured by government and private agencies into cancer research. Do you think any of this has brought tangible results in terms of preventing or treating cancer?*

A. Not really, because most investigators are still researching in accordance with the same old concept that cancer cells are the real problem, and that the destruction of those cells is the solution. Instead of focusing on killing cancer cells, which are merely a symptom of a systemic problem, research funds should be used to discover what is out of order with the human system as a whole. The research effort should be applied to what is causing the production of abnormal cells and designing methods to correct the dysfunction.

Q. *Do you believe that none of the research studies in the field of immunology has thrown any light on cancer that might be helpful in terms of the biorepair concept?*

A. No. It wasn't research that threw light on immunology. What did open up new thinking in that direction was the fact that transplants were being done—especially heart transplants—on a large scale. In order to avoid rejection of a foreign organ, the immune system had to be suppressed. As a result, immunosuppressive drugs had to be used. These are the same drugs that are used in chemotherapy. In using these drugs, doctors found there was a dramatic increase in cancer within the transplant patient population. This created an awareness that there was a vitally important link between the immune system and cancer.

By the way, I would like to add that there were people outside and within the medical establishment who were working independently on immunology research. I can list a number of individuals who were involved in the area of immunology research long before the cancer/immunity link was recognized. Among them were: Dr. Antonio Rottino of St. Vincent's Hospital in New York City, Dr. Isaac Djerassi at Catholic Mercy Medical Center in Philadelphia and Dr. Andrew Ivy of Illinois. Dr. Rottino's work is the basis of what is being done at the Burton Center in the Bahamas. Immunotherapy has not been used to its maximum because the medical community doesn't understand the physiology of immunotherapy well enough yet to feel comfortable depending on it. But if we are talking about the acceptance by researchers and oncologists of the role of the immunological system in defending the body against cancer and assisting in the cure, this has been acknowledged.

Q. *In your opinion, what would be the most productive direction in cancer research?*

A. An investigation to determine just where the biological breakdown that is responsible for the production of abnormal cells has taken place, then designing techniques to repair it efficiently. The system should develop noninvasive diagnostic tools, systems and mechanisms, and a whole-body approach to cancer treatment, rather than a fragmented one that aims at reducing the size of the tumor. It should protect the integrity of the body and avoid damage that would be impossible to overcome, repair, rebuild or detoxify. It should restore the host's healing ability to its optimum capability. Tumor reduction should be accomplished without harm to the integrity of the body by using techniques such as systemic thermotherapy. This would preserve the capability of achieving full recovery.

Q. *What should an individual do if cancer is detected?*

A. As I have been saying again and again, the individual has to investigate all the options that are open, and then make his or her decision. I know how hard it is to do that. But since the doctors often have to contend with controversies on what needs to be done, what you want to do is listen to all sides and then decide on the basis of your own thinking and feelings. Of course, it's easier for some people to submit to the doctor's choice of treatments, without having any responsibility for the decision. But stop and think that his or her decision—because of his or her obligation to offer the established protocols—may not always be right for you. I don't think you need to be afraid to participate in making the choice. In defense of doctors, let me add that I find most of them very cooperative, knowledgeable and compassionate.

Q. *How can one be certain that the physician is telling the cancer patient the truth about his or her condition?*

A. It is very painful for doctors to deal with cancer patients, especially when the problem may be too advanced for treatment. Doctors will often tell the patient what we call a "compassionate lie." They might appear to be busy, or they won't answer questions or else give vague answers. There is, however, a way to get information from the doctor—though some patients actually don't want to be told the truth. There is a Supreme Court decision to the effect that if a patient is offered treatments, he or she cannot make an "informed decision" unless he or she is given accurate information; therefore, tell your doctor you want to make an "informed decision" and he or she will give you all the information you need. Though the doctor may hesitate out of a sense of compassion to deliver the hard facts, I think it is better that the facts be given if the patient wants to know.

I know a patient who was given a prognosis of two months to two years to live due to a melanoma. He was told that even with a recommended leg amputation, he couldn't possibly live beyond two years. Well, that prognosis prompted him into investigating what could be done beyond the doctor's proposal. He started on Krebiozen, an immunotherapy program with Dr. Andrew Ivy, and the Kelley Metabolic Program. He never did have his leg amputated. That was more than twenty years ago. We need to know all the facts if we want to make an informed decision.

Q. *Is there any evidence that simply not treating a patient with traditional treatment modalities can actually increase the survival time?*

A. Dr. Hardin Jones, of Berkeley, CA, did some fine research, documented and published at the New York Academy of Sciences. He demonstrated that patients survived at least four times as long without treatment as with treatment, except in cases where there was an emergency. When there is a life-threatening body dysfunction, for example, it is urgent that the cancer receive attention first.

Q. *Does cancer spread because of surgery or a biopsy?*

A. It all depends on one's concept of cancer. If one believes that cancer is, in essence, nothing but the tumor—and that the whole body does not need to be repaired—then of course it could be assumed that cancer cells spread through surgery or biopsy. But if you accept the view that cancer has probably been developing within the whole system for a long time, that concept would not necessarily be accurate.

As one doctor with whom I shared a convention platform told me, cancer develops and spreads through the bloodstream, so that it makes no difference if surgery is done. The cancer cells actually have been reaching the tumor site through the bloodstream. This approach fits right into the biological concept of cancer—the whole system must be corrected, not merely the symptom.

Q. *My friend just had a baby who was born with cancer and none of the techniques for correcting diet or stress or anything else are applicable in this case. The doctors immediately started giving the baby chemotherapy. We are terrified about what can happen to the baby and wonder what kinds of alternatives there are.*

A. We never, under any circumstances, interfere with a doctor-patient relationship by urging the use of alternatives. There is no way in which we will tell an individual not to take chemotherapy, or whether or not to submit to radiation or surgery. The only thing we can do is give them information about the side effects that chemotherapy can produce or for instance, tell them if a small child's spine is radiated, there is a great likelihood that the spine will not grow normally.

Q. *Why do so many doctors give drugs so routinely—whether or not you need them?*

A. Your question makes certain assumptions that need to be examined carefully. In the first place, people have an unfortunate tendency to want treatment for the slightest sign of fever, the slightest sign of a cold, the slightest sign of illness, by immediately going to a doctor. Since you are seeking help, the doctor feels he has an obligation to provide treatment. A prominent physician, Dr. John Knowles of the Rockefeller Institute, made the statement at a medical convention that 90% of the patients going to a doctor would probably heal naturally—and only 10% actually need the doctor's help. If you visit a doctor for treatment, he feels obliged to treat you. He assumes that is the reason for the visit. He cannot take the risk that the condition will be neglected and worsen and he will be held responsible. For the most part, this is what people expect and want unless the doctor is told that the visit is just to have his professional opinion.

On occasion you might run into a doctor who was trained somewhat differently a long time ago, and he or she may say to you, "Why don't you wait a day or so? Take some tea, rest and see what happens." But this is rare today because of the threat of a malpractice suit. By and large, a doctor is going to serve you by giving you some medication if it is indicated—and rightfully so, according to his training. A doctor-patient relationship should be a partnership. If you allow him or her to make the entire determination, by not participating in the decision, you are equally responsible. It is not his or her role to be entirely responsible for the decision—unless you give it to the doctor. It is not his or her place to tell you to use more natural healing, or to suggest that you wait for the illness to alleviate itself. If you choose to go to a doctor, you must be prepared for conventional treatments.

What I am talking about is the participation of the individual in his or her own medical care. This doesn't mean that one has to refuse to listen to the doctor's advice. Not at all. It does mean, however, that one ought to be an intelligent medical consumer, know what to look for, and use the doctor's professional skills in a partnership arrangement.

Nutrition

Q. *I understand how important raw vegetables are to a proper diet. But what if one has difficulty using vegetables in the raw state?*

A. Some people who suffer from ulcers or colitis, or who have had intestinal surgery, do have problems eating raw vegetables. When this is the case, one can liquefy the vegetables by using a juice extractor. This will separate the pulp from the liquid. When you do this, you are getting the nutritional value of the vegetables, the rest being discardable pulp. The pulp is beneficial roughage for colon cleansing and can be obtained from other sources. Another method is to use a blender or food processor. Occasionally, people complain that eating raw vegetables causes a great deal of gas. Usually, it's not the vegetables that are to blame, since these are excellent quality materials that the body needs. Sometimes, however, the vegetables begin to loosen the gummy mucous that has coated the villi along the intestinal wall. When these putrefied materials start to flow, they will cause gas. People who have this problem may call it an allergy to a particular food. But if the diet is changed slowly, starting with cooked vegetables and gradually adding raw, one may find that eventually the body will be able to utilize the higher quality material without generating gas.

Q. *Are there any particular fruits or vegetables that are healthier than others?*

A. One should include a wide variety of fruits and vegetables in the diet. There is nothing that shows us that we should have a preference for one kind of food over another—whether it is citrus fruits or spinach as touted by industry sources. But if you overuse vegetables which contain oxalic acid, such as spinach, beets and Swiss chard, they will drain the body of calcium, one of our most important elements, as the body needs calcium for a host of body functions. There is no difficulty if foods are used in moderation.

Q. *What nutritional role do foods such as parsley and watercress play?*

A. These foods fall more into the area of herbs than vegetables. As such, they are helpful and flavorful.

I would like to comment about herbs in general. Some people assume that just because they are botanicals, all are safe substances that can be used on an unlimited basis. Many of the herbals were our original medicines and listed in the medical pharmacopeia. They should still be considered as such. They do not have the harmful aspect of chemical medicine, they usually have no lasting side effects or deprive the body of essentials as chemical pharmaceuticals do, and they accomplish their function as a safer kind of medicine. So, certainly, it would be useful to go back to Nature's herbal remedies. But we must be more discriminating and use these natural elements in an intelligent fashion. Also, a differentiation ought to be made between medicinal herbs (which should be treated with caution) and the culinary herbs or herbal teas, which can be a sound part of the daily dietary program, and are an adventure in various tastes.

Q. *The outer skins and leaves of fruits and vegetables contain some valuable food elements. Yet this is exactly where you would expect the highest concentration of chemical residues. Would you, therefore, remove the outer elements and lose some of its nutrients, or rather eat the entire foods after washing them, in the hope that somehow the better nutrition will balance out the harmful chemicals?*

A. The skin may be too loaded with dangerous chemical residues. It is better to peel or remove the outer skins, and carefully wash other vegetables to get rid of as much of the remaining contaminants as possible. Unfortunately, we are caught in a less than perfect environment.

Q. *Is a low-protein diet a sensible nutritional regime for a cancer patient?*

A. I don't think there is any quarrel at this time that low protein is a better yardstick—not only for cancer patients but for all individuals. The government criterion for daily protein intake is 46 grams for a woman and 56 grams for a man. I believe this measurement should be based on height and weight; a small woman and a small man should use the 46 grams and a large woman and man should use 56 grams. There are some instances, however, when the cancer patient is not able to metabolize protein well enough to eat even the required amount of protein. In these cases, one can take proteolytic enzymes to help metabolize the protein.

Dr. Max Gerson's system was to remove protein entirely from his patient's diet at the start of treatment, except for liver juice. He reintroduced protein, usually cottage cheese, (since protein is an essential nutrient for cell production) after about five or six weeks. He limited the protein initially in the belief that there are occasions when protein must be reduced for a period of time in order to give the body a chance to begin its rebalancing process. Ordinarily, however, healthy bodily maintenance includes sufficient protein just as it requires other nutrients.

Q. *You often hear or read in health circles that proteins should be taken in certain combinations, such as rice and beans, to give you the complete protein. Is it true that you can't get the whole protein except in combination?*

A. The people who talk about creating complete proteins from rice and beans are individuals who are vegetarians, striving to get all of the required amino acids in one meal. There is no substantial evidence that if an individual eats at different times of the day but gets all of the amino acids the body requires, that there is any danger at all. People do not have to make certain that each dish is so arranged that it has to have all of the required amino acids at one time. The body will metabolize the amino acids that it needs if they are eaten in the course of a day. Nature has a special wisdom; it doesn't create food to cause harm.

Q. *Should cancer patients eat meat?*

A. I have already talked about meat as a source of protein. Some cancer patients must have some meat, just as most cancer-free individuals *require this food.* Evidently, over generations of meat-eating ancestors, the body, in its effort to maintain health, has adapted to its environment and therefore meat has become a requirement. The confusion lies in the fact that we do not require a huge amount of meat, nor do we require all of our protein from flesh foods. There is protein in such foods as nuts, beans and avocados—and even a little in vegetables and fruits.

Q. *Are eggs and cheese essential for the cancer patient?*

A. I don't think that anyone can say that they are essential or not essential for any particular individual but they are a good form of protein, providing they are organic. The amount of protein has to be decided on an individualized basis.

Q. *Would it be helpful for a cancer patient to change over to a vegetarian diet under the supervision of a competent practitioner?*

A. Not necessarily. The only diet that is helpful is the one that is relevant to any particular human system. Some people can be on a vegetarian diet, some cannot. Unfortunately, many young people today have adopted a vegetarian diet, indiscriminately, under the assumption that a vegetarian diet is ideal. Not only is this untrue, but it may actually play havoc with the individual's health if it is inapplicable to their body chemistry.

There is another matter that has to be cleared up about vegetarianism. There is in fact no single vegetarian diet. There is lacto-vegetarian, ovo-vegetarian, lacto-ovo-vegetarian, the Hygienist system, and others. The only thing in common is that they use no flesh protein. Some vegetarian diets can include canned food, processed food, junk foods, fried food and pastries and so forth. So you can see that vegetarianism is not at all synonymous with good health.

Q. *Everyone knows how difficult it is to purchase all our products organically. What is a patient to do if he can't find sufficient fruits and vegetables that are uncontaminated, and has to use sprayed or otherwise chemicalized foods?*

A. Certainly, the more organic foods that one can buy, the less the body is subjected to toxic chemicals, especially since contaminated foods could have created the health problem in the first place. The more you can avoid unwholesome foods, the easier it is to recover one's health. Unfortunately, today there is no way to eliminate contaminated foods altogether and still have a balanced dietary program in which the body gets all of its requirements. Therefore, one should try to get as many organic foods as possible, and only shop outside of the organic market when it is necessary to balance one's nutritional needs.

Q. *Many foods in the supermarket carry the words "all natural" on the label. Is this a sign of nutritional progress, or is it simply another advertising hook to entice the buyer?*

A. I think that is progress in so far as it recognizes that people are looking for more natural foods, and it may not be a marketing trick at all on the part of the manufacturer. That doesn't mean, however, that one can accept without question the terminology used for every product. One must always ask: What do they mean in this instance by "all natural?" Of course, there is no clear-cut government standard of measurement. The manufacturer could in all truth be presenting natural materials, but that is no reason to assume that each manufacturer's criterion for natural is the same. The value system of the Food and Drug Administration is that everything is natural, even chemicals. I don't want to discredit the manufacturer's desire to meet the consumers' demands for a higher quality food, but I prefer to use the term "organic" rather than natural. And I would define organic food as material that is whole rather than fragmented, has not gone through any refining process, contains no chemical additives, and is grown on soil without chemical pesticides. Meanwhile, it would be a good idea for the consumer to examine the label carefully for the contents.

Q. *Is the taking of raw bran daily a good form of roughage?*

A. No. A better form of roughage is to use whole grains, raw vegetables and fruits. When you take bran, it certainly does provide additional roughage, and has been known to initiate better colon activity, but you are also taking a food material which is not in its whole form. It is a fragmented food, just as wheat without its hull is not a whole food. The hull without its kernel is not a whole grain. Important food elements are therefore missing so that it is no longer synergistic.

Q. *Do you see any value in the practice of using protein powder which is available in health food stores?*

A. No. There is no need for protein powder. It is preferable to get protein through the use of protein foods. I think the use of protein powder is related to a fad in the assumption that high protein is the most wholesome kind of diet—which it is not. Feeding the body its required amount of protein is what makes a healthful diet. The proper balanced diet includes neither deficiency nor overload.

Q. *Why is clabbered milk considered so healthful?*

A. First of all, it's a naturally soured milk, which means that healthy bacteria in the milk have gone to work to start the digestive process. It becomes a more healthful food than sweet milk, because as you know, adults do not have the enzyme, lactase, needed to digest sweet milk. Babies have this enzyme, but in a natural environment it is no longer needed after a baby has been weaned. Nature therefore arranges for the production of this enzyme to wane. Clabbered milk, however, can be digested easily because the predigestion process has already taken place. Clabbered milk also provides good intestinal flora to replace flora that might be destroyed by preservatives added to the food or antibiotics.

Supplements

Q. *When are digestive enzyme supplements indicated?*

A. Enzymes are used therapeutically in a biorepair program to ensure that food is competently metabolized. Individuals who have eaten poorly for a long period of time might have weakened their enzymatic function ergo, need supplementary enzymes, possibly for the rest of their lives, to help digest their food. They may have simply worn out the ability of the digestive organs to supply adequate secretions for good enzymatic function. Enzyme supplements are particularly important with cooked foods, as heat destroys enzymes. A tablet may contain a wide range of useful enzymes such as: pancrease, amylase, cellulase, lipase, and hydrochloric acid. It should not have a color coating nor be enteric coated. Enteric coating is protein. If protein metabolism is poor, the coating may not be eliminated sufficiently, so the tablet may pass through the system without being used competently.

It's simple to include supplementary enzymes if needed. The amount can be started at the minimum level and increase as indicated based on the results. In my own situation, I was told that my digestive system was not up to par, and that I would have to take enzymes for the rest of my life as a result of years of poor eating habits. I had to determine what my need was, and I found that I don't have to take more than one with each meal. We all have our unique constitution to work with, our own functional weaknesses, and therefore, our own specific supplementary needs.

Q. *What do you think of Dr. Linus Pauling's claim that large doses of vitamin C are beneficial to patients with cancer?*

A. There is an opposite view that megadoses of vitamin C or megadoses of any one vitamin can ultimately burn out the enzymes needed for metabolism and, therefore, imbalance body chemistry, so high doses become a problem. There is always the danger that when one uses materials in such excessive quantities, a metabolic imbalance will be created. Actually, from my point of view, megadoses of vitamin C, or any therapy focused specifically on attacking the tumor, is just another variation on the conventional medical model which ultimately fails because it doesn't restore normal cell production. Dr. Pauling, who probably did more to promote vitamin C than anyone else, died of prostate cancer even though he probably took his own advice and used vitamin C in megadoses.

Q. *What is the distinction between natural vitamin E and a synthetic form?*

A. I will relate a story that might explain this difference in more practical terms. I asked Alan Nitler, M.D., a very fine nutritionist, to speak before a group of doctors. He reported that he had a heart patient whom he had put on 200-400 mgs of vitamin E, as recommended by a Dr. Shute, which though not synthetic, is nevertheless a processed form of the vitamin. He gave the patient somewhere between 800 and 1200 milligrams a day. In measuring this patient with a cardiogram, he found that he was not getting positive results. He then decided to use wheat germ oil—which is of course a more natural substance, closer to a biological material. He gave 600 milligrams by the teaspoonful. That form of vitamin E was utilized much more effectively by the body, achieving good results. This situation with vitamin E should be used and applied to other nutritional substances—it doesn't have to be limited to vitamin E alone.

Dr. Royal Lee, one of the early pioneers to study natural supplements in depth, developed a heart-measuring device which is different from what is ordinarily used. The company he founded, Standard Process Laboratories, produces a tablet which contains only 2 milligrams of vitamin E. *It is an all-natural supplement.* When he used his heart-measuring device on patients taking his low-potency 2 mg tablet of all-natural E and compared it with those taking high-potency processed E, the response with the 2 mg tablet of natural vitamin E was superior. These are experiences I am personally aware of which provide strong evidence of the merit of natural versus synthetic. Consider the fact, in this instance, that the 2 milligram dosage was found to be more effective than the 800-1200 milligrams that Dr. Shute had recommended.

Q. *Would you care to comment on Laetrile?*

A. My position on Laetrile, which is derived from apricot kernels, has changed from the one which I originally held. Years ago a form of Laetrile was used which was only 65% refined. As more people sought Laetrile, more companies manufactured it. Most of these suppliers thought that refining the apricot kernels about 95% was an improvement. Many of us in the health movement know that a natural substance when overrefined becomes somewhat devitalized. I think this is what happened to Laetrile. In my opinion it might be better to use the apricot kernels.

Detoxification

Q. *How can individuals who utilize enemas and colonics regularly be certain that they are not depleting their intestinal systems of the needed "friendly" bacteria? I know that you recommend some form of fermented food, but some so-called wholistic practitioners don't think we should use enemas too often, or even at all.*

A. They would be right if the colon were clean and healthy, with good muscle tone. Colon cleansing is designed to help the colon eliminate its waste and clear out encrusted waste that has adhered to the colon wall, until it can function more efficiently without help. In many instances the colon muscles have become inefficient because the encrusted feces blocks muscle activity. The water from the enema gradually cleans the colon and allows the muscles to be reactivated. Some individuals may be able to get away without using enemas as part of the detoxification procedures, but it is very rare. My position is that it is better to take an enema for the rest of one's life, if that becomes necessary, than to risk failing to achieve complete recovery from a health problem.

Q. *Do you feel, as it is so often claimed, that an exclusive grapefruit juice diet is excellent for cleansing purposes?*

A. Perhaps. Alan Nittler, M.D., liked to put his patients on a diet of two fruits for two weeks for detoxification. Incidentally, using a mono-food as a cleansing system need not be restricted to grapefruit. Watermelon or any other fruit can be used for a period of two weeks or more, but it should be supervised by someone competent. There is always the risk, if one does it alone, that the juices will stimulate some heavy reactions. The individual may get to the point where the toxins that are released move too rapidly from the cells—where they have been stored—to the bloodstream. Without understanding the nature of toxicity in the bloodstream, the symptoms can be very distressing.

Q. *Would you suggest a sauna as a means of inducing perspiration, or is this technique too taxing for a cancer patient?*

A. Any procedure that will help bring some of the toxins to the surface for elimination is good. And certainly the skin is one of the avenues by which the body rids itself of waste.

Q. *Do you think the product comfrey/pepsin is useful for waste elimination?*

A. That is not the purpose of comfrey/pepsin. Pepsin is used to clean the intestinal wall of the gummy coating on the villi which is limiting absorption of nutrients into the bloodstream. Since comfrey is mucilaginous, by combining the pepsin to it, the pepsin adheres to the intestinal wall allowing it to dissolve the gummy accumulation. Comfrey/pepsin should not be a permanent part of supplement intake as the intestines require a mucous coating. As soon as it has completed its work, the comfrey/pepsin should be discontinued.

Q. *Is there a good natural diuretic?*

A. Yes, asparagus and watermelon act as good diuretics. There are also herbal diuretics.

Q. *You mention that it is important to get some of the wastes out of the lymphatic system. Can you suggest some of the techniques that can help in this regard?*

A. Keeping the lymphatic system from being clogged is very important. Some of the best ways to do this is through exercise, lymphatic massage, adding a small quantity of beets to juice and using the bouncer, which is like a mini trampoline. Detoxification is important, especially the procedure that was originally in the book, *Fresh Vegetable and Fruit Juices*, by Norman Walker.

Diagnostic Procedures

Q. *What are your thoughts about mammography when used as a routine technique?*

A. Dr. John C. Bailar III, when he was with the National Cancer Institute, made a public statement about the harm of routine mammography. Women were having this procedure done once a year and many of them twice a year. He said that the effects were cumulative and could be carcinogenic. Of course, there was some controversy with the radiologists, who said that it was not harmful.

Some years ago, the Surgeon General came to the conclusion that mammography used routinely to detect cancer should not be done. The official compromise was that women under 45 should not resort to yearly x-rays, while women over 45 should. In other words, if it was going to be cumulative, one could get by without apparent adverse effects for twenty or thirty years. I suppose the reasoning is that a woman over 45 is approaching a time of her life when cancer is more common.

Under these circumstances, I don't think we need authorities to set such standards for us. It doesn't mean that the x-rays are less harmful for the over-45 and more harmful for the under-45 section of the population.

Today, thankfully, the Food and Drug Administration is definitely saying that one should limit the use of x-rays and keep an accurate record of x-rays taken. When the FDA arrives at the point where they participate in warning against x-rays, you had better accept the fact that there is a danger involved in overexposure.

Q. *If mammography is not a safe detection technique, what is?*

A. I would like to suggest a system called thermography. It is based on the principle that cancer cells are hotter than normal cells. Special equipment is used to measure the heat of the cells. You get a more accurate determination of trouble with this device than you do with x-rays. X-rays are a very inconclusive diagnostic procedure; they do not always produce a clear image. But when thermography shows that heat is present, it suggests that further evaluation is indicated. The cells are not necessarily malignant—they could be inflamed instead. It does indicate, at least, whether or not there is a problem, without using offensive x-rays. Though it is usually limited to diagnosis of breast cancer, I am told that thermography can be used to detect any kind of "soft" cancer of internal organs such as the liver or pancreas. In any event, one can submit yearly or even more often to this form of diagnosis without a qualm. Although there are some blood tests for cancer, they are usually used to monitor a patient instead of for diagnosis. There is a higher inaccuracy rate with those techniques.

Q. *Is there any way to avoid a barium enema in a situation where they have to diagnose a colon problem?*

A. Yes, a colonoscope can be used safely in lieu of a barium enema, so that one can avoid some x-ray exposure and barium. The colonoscope is a flexible fiber-optic tube that is used extensively these days. It was first perfected by Dr. Hiromi Shinya, and originally, you had to go to him if you wanted this form of diagnosis. Now it is available elsewhere. The tube is placed into the colon, and because of its flexibility, reaches across the transverse area.

Of course, today colonoscopy has become the standard technique and barium enemas are rarely used. The colonoscope has a diamond-shaped wire attached to it, so that if there is a polyp in the colon and it is attached on a threadlike filament, it can be snipped off and biopsied. Years ago, if polyps existed in the transverse area, the only way to get them out was through a surgical procedure.

Psychological and Physical Factors

Q. *As one who has been under extreme stress for a long time, I am concerned with Dr. Selye's statement that chronic stress could do permanent damage to the endocrine system. Do you agree with this?*

A. Though I cannot argue with Dr. Selye's excellent research, I would have to accept with some reservation the statement that chronic stress can cause permanent damage to the endocrine system. A number of other unhealthful conditions—and degenerative diseases—have also been considered irreversible. Yet, from my experience with patients who have used the biological approach to repair, I know this is not necessarily so. The body has powerful repair capability when given the right conditions. For example, I am aware of patients with epilepsy, high blood pressure, diabetes, deafness, macular degeneration, arthritis—and of course cancer—who were able to restore their body chemistry back to normal balance. So you see what can be done if one undergoes a sound and individually-tailored biorepair program. I would, therefore, be inclined to lean towards the conclusion that the body can make the necessary correction if it is given the right conditions.

Q. *Despite the fact that I have been on a biofeedback program, under the supervision of an expert, I have been unable to control or even reduce my chronic stress. Can you suggest why this form of stress management is not helping me?*

A. It may be that in your particular situation, the cause of the stress has not been determined and corrected, so that benefit is only temporary. Biofeedback does help to provide relief from the impact of stress on body function.

Q. *Does one have to experience symptoms such as pains in the jaw, spasms, headaches or backaches to be suffering from TMJ misalignment?*

A. Not necessarily. A displaced TMJ can be the root cause of any number of other health problems, including chronic tension, poor digestion, and an inability of the spine to hold to a proper alignment. The wisest course is to have the TMJ checked by a dentist who is knowledgeable in TMJ.

Q. *Would you consider isometrics a good form of exercise for cancer patients?*

A. Absolutely. Isometrics are exercises that strengthen muscles, not through strenuous activity, but by pitting one part of the body against another without undue pressure. For example, pushing the fist of one hand against the palm of another would be considered isometric.

There are other good exercises such as yoga-type postures, walking and gentle stretching movements. These are preferable to activities which are overly vigorous. In other words, the aim is to keep the muscles limber and toned, but not overdeveloped, stressed or strained. Isometrics meet this exercise requirement.

Cancer-Inducing Agents

Q. *Do you believe there is a link between cancer and fluoridated water?*

A. This link has been well established. Dr. John Yiammouyiannis, a scientist who investigated the connection between fluoridated water and cancer, was an extremely able biochemist—I knew him very well. He was very careful in his research, and tried to cover every aspect of fluoridation, so that there was no way to discredit his statistics. Other scientists have added their voices to claim the carcinogenicity of fluoride. We must understand that fluorides are toxic substances. Whether it is fluoride or any other toxic substance, we must do our best to avoid ingesting them because of their cumulative effect. And when toxins accumulate, you never know what health breakdown will result.

Q. *Is there anything that can be done to reduce the dangers of chemical contamination when one works in a factory where these substances are present in the environment?*

A. Hopefully, the Occupational Safety and Health Administration's (OSHA) current guidelines can help control exposure to carcinogens and other dangerous pollutants. Frankly, however, despite the conscious effort of our government agencies, these regulations are far from adequate in protecting workers from the effects of toxic materials. Though it is not practical for most people to do so, the best strategy under those circumstances is to find other employment. If that is impossible, then, one should eat healthfully, exercise, get fresh air, rest adequately, and reduce stress. In other words, build host resistance.

Q. *Why doesn't our government do more testing of chemicals for their possible carcinogenic effects?*

A. Testing chemicals is a very slow and expensive process. The government agencies responsible for testing can't go through more than a few carcinogenic testing procedures at a time. When one considers the vast amount of chemicals already being used industrially, and the hundreds of new ones that are introduced each year, you can see the immensity of the problem. In any case, the current testing techniques are not the best anyway, because they are done animal systems, which function differently from human systems. I don't believe they reach sound conclusions in the long run. My own position is that there should be nothing toxic allowed, whether in the atmosphere, the work environment, food or water. These substances do not have to be carcinogenic to be dangerous. The fact that they are toxic means that they are biologically unsound and therefore do not suit the human system. Chemicals that do not appear to be carcinogenic can cause a biochemical breakdown when they become cumulative or possibly, may become carcinogenic when combined with other chemicals in the environment.

Q. *My dentist thinks I need a full series of x-rays, even though I had this done about a year ago. He dismisses my arguments that it might be harmful by pointing out that the amount of x-ray exposure on his new machine is equivalent to less than half an hour's exposure to the sun. How do I answer his arguments?*

A. I would not answer; I would not argue; I would simply not subject myself to routine x-rays. I would only allow the minimum and only when necessary. I want to suggest that people read John W. Goffman, M.D.'s important book *Radiation and Human Health,* on the dangers of x-rays. He too takes the position that x-rays are sometimes necessary, but he warns against their indiscriminate use, and the dangers to the human system. If you have a dental problem, let the doctor first determine what it is with his pick, as they did years ago. If that doesn't work, and you must have an x-ray, let him x-ray the one tooth only, not routinely the whole mouth.

Miscellaneous

Q. *How do you differentiate between the symptoms that arise during the repair process and legitimate health problems?*

A. Actually, it is extremely difficult to tell whether they are symptoms of ill health or that the body is going through a healing phase. I can only tell you how I would deal with the situation myself. I would allow the reactions—or the flare-ups, as they are sometimes called—to run their course for a period of time. After I had waited for a time and gone through a detoxifying procedure and found that I was improving, I would then know that it was actually a healing phase that had caused the symptoms. This would be an indication that the body was taking care of its condition. If, however, the symptoms do not improve and gradually become worse, then it is probably a disease progression and steps should be taken to reevaluate the program.

Q. *There is currently a good deal of controversy about inoculating school children. How do you feel about this?*

A. I would classify inoculations as another violation of the human system and interfering with Nature's processes. A healthy system can withstand childhood diseases, and once young people go through them, the immune system is stronger. In other words, the body has made the most of what Nature has designed.

I don't believe that inoculation should be mandated by legislative bodies. The decision ought to be based on freedom of choice. There are some parents following different health concepts who feel their children don't require inoculation as they have good host resistance, and their doctors concur. Their feelings should be honored. Nor do I believe that the reverse should take place, where parents are told that no one should be allowed inoculations.

There is another consideration that has to be thought about. The argument is often made that all children should be inoculated, presumably because if some children are not inoculated, others will be in danger. But this is not a valid assumption. If they stopped to think about it and, indeed feel inoculations are protective, they would realize that children who are not inoculated in no way should be able to threaten those who have been inoculated. Many children, for example, have had polio, and not been crippled by it at all, and certainly have not passed along the disease to others.

Q. *The claim is sometimes made that the process by which water is distilled removes all of the minerals. If this is so, how can we replace those minerals when we use distilled water?*

A. This is an argument that keeps raging over and over again. Dr. Norman Walker, who can be considered an authority on the use of distilled water, believed that minerals in spring, well or tap water are inorganic and will not be absorbed well by the body. He has written that water that contains inorganic minerals actually starts the ageing process. Dr. Walker died at the age of 117 after a lifetime use of distilled water. That must tell us something.

Nature converts minerals derived from plants into organic materials which are readily absorbable. This is where one gets minerals. People who are trying to derive the greatest benefit from the repair system should drink distilled water, because it is not contaminated with chemicals, and is our safest source for water. The greater concern about water, other than distilled water, is contaminants in spring water coming from the polluted underground rivers (aquifers).

Q. *Does the body's immunity consist of its antibodies, or is it a generalized response against disease?*

A. The immune defenses are actually made up of a number of entities. These include the lymphatics, the thymus gland, the liver, and the waste elimination system. I should add that, to the degree that one repairs the dysfunction of the body as a whole, one also improves the effectiveness of the entire immune defenses.

Q. *For those of us who are relatively healthy and don't have cancer, what advice would you give us to help maintain our health?*

A. First of all, we have to do whatever we can to see that we are not ingesting carcinogens and other pollutants that are added to our food and water supply. The quantities may be small, but sometimes one uses many foods with the same additives and in this way ingests more than the tolerable dose. Your water is very important, too. It should be distilled in order to have the safest supply. Wells and aquifers are too polluted to be trusted and some of the chemicals cannot be detected with the present technical equipment. The hardest thing to control is the air, but if other factors are corrected, the body will be better able to tolerate this singular abuse.

The food you eat should be balanced, and much of it should be raw, so that you get the benefit of all the natural nutrients, without destruction of enzymes from heat and loss of minerals thrown out with the cooking water. Protein intake should be on the low side and come from sources that do not contain carcinogenic hormones, antibiotics or from animals fed rendered feed. Complex carbohydrates, such as potatoes, whole grains, and beans, are very nourishing, too, and can be prepared simply so as to retain all of their food value. A good ferment is also appropriate in order to maintain "friendly" flora in case there are preservatives in the food. The ferment can be yogurt, good quality sauerkraut, fermented juices or similar products. Even cheeses have the kind of bacteria needed to maintain beneficial intestinal flora.

This is a very general idea of a healthful diet. In addition, exercise, rest and relaxation, and a positive mental attitude have to be part of one's lifestyle, as well as active waste elimination. I have dealt with all of these elements before, but I think they bear repeating—and keeping in mind—for everyone who wants to do the most that is possible to assure continuing good health and cancer prevention.

Conclusion

The incidence of cancer continues to rise at an alarming rate. Unfortunately, it is impossible to completely protect yourself against the carcinogenic elements that exist in our environment. But there is much we can do to avoid being totally inundated with the enormous amount of toxic substances in our food and water. It is also useful to remember that Nature has provided a great capability for the body to repair itself, provided that biological integrity (host resistance) is achieved. It is vital that we develop and maintain a level of strong host resistance in the fight against cancer.

Healthy cell production is our goal, instead of cell destruction. The focus of conventional cancer treatment is cell destruction. The system doesn't heal or restore, therefore, it usually only buys time. You must also consider that not all alternative therapies are safe and biologically sound. When examining your options, please stop and ask yourself *"Does this approach focus on the enhancement and maintainance of host integrity?"*

My intention is not to promote one treatment over another, or to discredit conventional oncologists. Each case is different and each case should be individualized. Each individual should also take responsibility for his or her decisions, preferably with professional or knowledgeable guidance.

I have dedicated over thirty years of my life to FACT, a nonprofit organization dedicated to a different concept of cancer and cancer treatment. I have gathered vast experience and knowledge from practitioners and patients that have achieved success through the use of biologically sound therapies. Constantly, new treatments and supplements pop up, claiming to be the cure for cancer. Please remember that there is no magic potion. The whole body must be treated, and biological integrity must be preserved. I am confident that through greater awareness of biologically sound systems to effect a biorepair, the devastation of cancer can be controlled.

The Foundation for Advancement in Cancer Therapy is available to cancer patients to provide information collected through our thirty years of experience. FACT is available to provide guidance in making decisions in choosing a therapy, to offer information about resourses, and to respond to a myriad of miscellaneous needs.

Bibliography

Bieler, Henry. *Food Is Your Best Medicine*. New York: Ballantine Books, 1990.

Cousins, Norman. *Anatomy of an Illness as Perceived by the Patient*. New York: Bantam Books, 1986.

Dement, William and Christopher Vaughn. *The Promise of Sleep*. New York: Delacorte Press, 1999.

Fagin, Dan, Marianne Lavelle and Center for Public Integrity. *Toxic Deception: How the Chemical Industry Manipulates Science, Bends the Law, and Endangers Your Health*. Monroe: Common Courage Press, 1999.

Ford Heritage. *Composition and Facts About Foods*. Mokelumne Hill: Health Research, 1971.

Gerson, Max. *A Cancer Therapy: Results of Fifty Cases and the Cure of Advanced Cancer*. San Diego: Gerson Institute, 1997.

Goffman, John. *Radiation and Human Health*. San Francisco: Sierra Club Books, 1981.

Greenfield, Louise. *Cancer Overcome By Diet*. Louise Greenfield, 1987.

Hay, William Howard. *How to Always Be Well*. c.1930 (out-of-print, reissued by FACT)

Howell, Edward. *Enzyme Nutrition*. Wayne: Avery, 1985.

Hoxsey, Harry. *You Don't Have to Die*. Los Angeles: Cancer Book House, 1985.

Hunsberger, Eydie May. *How I Conquered Cancer Naturally*. Garden City Park: Avery, 1992.

Jensen, Bernard. *A New Lifestyle for Health and Happiness.* Escondido: Bernard Jensen International, 1980.

Jensen, Bernard. *Tissue Cleansing Through Bowel Management.* Escondido: Bernard Jensen International, 1981.

Kelley, William Donald. *One Answer to Cancer.* Mineral Wells: Cancer Coalition, 1997.

Lane, Sir William Arbuthnot. *The Prevention of the Diseases Peculiar to Civilization.* (out-of-print, reissued by FACT, 1981)

Lee, John. *Natural Progesterone.* Oxfordshire: Jon Carpenter Publishing, 1999.

Levine, Barbara H. *Your Body Believes Every Word You Say.* Fairfield: WordsWork Press, 2000.

Ott, John. *Health and Light: The Effects of Natural and Artificial Light on Man and Other Living Things.* Alpharetta: Ariel Press, 2000.

Physicians' Desk Reference for Herbal Medicines. Montvale: Medical Economics, 2000.

Sedlacek, Keith and Matthew Culligan. *How to Avoid Stress Before It Kills You.* New York: Gramercy Publishing, 1980.

Selye, Hans. *Stress Without Distress.* Philadelphia: Lippincott, Williams and Wilkins, 1974.

Sokosh, Doris. *Triumph Over Cancer: My Recipe for Recovery.* New York: FACT, 1997.

Tilden, John. *Toxemia Explained: The True Interpretation of the Cause of Disease.* Belle Fourche: Kessinger Publishing, 1997.

Waerland, Are. *Health Is Your Birthright.* Bern: Humata Publications.

Walker, Norman. *Fresh Vegetable and Fruit Juices.* Prescott: Norwalk Press, 1981.

Walker, Norman. *Vegetarian Guide to Diet & Salad.* Prescott: Norwalk Press, 1995.

Index

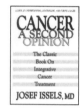
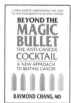

A WORD ABOUT F.A.C.T.

For over forty years, the Foundation for Advancement in Cancer Therapy (F.A.C.T.), a non-profit 501(c)(3) organization, has acted as a consumer advocacy group, educating cancer patients about alternative therapies and their rights as patients.

Although traditional medical groups and government agencies have often ignored or disregarded the groundbreaking work of many integrative medical researchers, F.A.C.T. has provided these pioneers with a platform to be heard. The foundation's intention has never been to discredit conventional medicine, but rather to scrutinize the alternative therapies, and then make the information available. In this way, cancer patients and their families can make informed, responsible decisions regarding treatment options.

Alternative medicine has made substantial headway into the realm of traditional medical services, but there still remains a major gap in the availability of information on nontoxic, noninvasive treatments. Ruth Sackman, Founder and former President of F.A.C.T., wrote *Rethinking Cancer* to meet this challenge and answer the many questions posed by today's growing number of cancer patients. *Rethinking Cancer* supplies pertinent information on a wide variety of topics, including the primary role of nutrition and detoxification in healing, how to repair the body's biological breakdowns, and ways to control one's own psychological influences on health. Drawing upon the experience of researchers worldwide, as well as the feedback of thousands of patients who have contacted F.A.C.T. over the years, *Rethinking Cancer* offers specific advice on dealing with and preventing the disease.

The F.A.C.T. website, www.rethinkingcancer.com provides a vast library of resources, ranging from articles and audio presentations to biorepair studies, as well as a practitioner directory. The Foundation has also created an informative educational film called *Rethinking Cancer*, which is available as a DVD and makes an excellent companion to the book. It is available at www.rethinkingcancer.com.

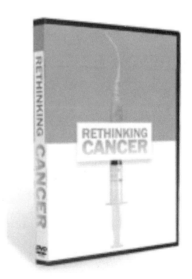

$19.95
ISBN 8 20360 13899 7
Running time: 56 minutes